BUGLE NOTES

WORDS OF ENCOURAGEMENT TO A MEDICAL STAFF

Andrew S. Lamb, MD

Contents

ABOUT THE AUTHOR

Dr. Andrew (Andy) Lamb is a board-certified Internal Medicine physician. A 1977 graduate of the United States Military Academy at West Point, he served 3 years on active duty in Germany before attending the University of Alabama in Birmingham School of Medicine on an Army Health Professions Scholarship. He graduated in 1984 and subsequently completed his residency in Internal Medicine in 1987 at Dwight D. Eisenhower Army Medical Center in Augusta, Georgia. He then served five years as an internist at Blanchfield Army Community Hospital, Ft Campbell, Kentucky, where he was also the Chief of Internal Medicine. In 1990, he deployed to Saudi Arabia as Chief of Medicine for the 86th Evacuation Hospital in support of the 101st Air Assault Division during Operation Desert Storm. He was awarded the Bronze Star for his service there.

In 1992, he left the Army and entered private practice with the Kernodle Clinic in Burlington, NC where he remained for 22 years. His life has been one of leadership and service. He has held numerous leadership positions to include President of Kernodle Clinic, Chief of Medicine, Alamance Regional Medical Center, and Chief of Staff, Alamance Regional Medical Center. In 2014, he was selected as the first Vice President of Medical Affairs with Cone Health – ARMC, a senior executive physician leadership position. He serves as the co-Medical Director of the Elon University Department of Physician Assistant Studies. He has taught medical students, physician assistants, and nurse practitioner students for nearly 30 years. Finally, Dr. Lamb is a team leader for faith-based medical missions throughout the world. Thus far, he has led 50 missions since 2000. His passion is investing in, teaching, encouraging, and mentoring others.

He is an avid fly fisherman and ties his own flies and makes fly rods. He enjoys backpacking and camping (combined with fly fishing!) as well as sports (he played baseball at West Point and coached youth baseball for nearly 20 years), reading, writing, and a good bourbon and cigar!

INTRODUCTION

In November 2000, I embarked on my first medical mission to a tiny, remote village high in the mountains of Guatemala. I went there for a number of reasons. Of course, one of them being that I wanted to help medically any way I could, but the reality was that the adventure, travel, and experiences of a new culture were my main motivations. Although this was a Christian-based mission, my primary motivations were personal. I returned home after an extremely busy and exhausting week only to be humbled by the kindness, generosity, and appreciation of those we served. They were always so nice and appreciative despite the great needs they had and the hardships they faced every day. I realized that the mission was not at all about me; it was far from that! It was all about God and loving and serving His creatures for Him. I had seen pictures and news clips of the overwhelming need that much of the world faces, but I had never experienced it firsthand. The need had never been personal to me, but now it was, and finally, it became my reality.

I continue to lead missions, and with each one, I learn even more about myself. Unexpectedly, I discovered how much I loved investing in, teaching, encouraging, and mentoring those who came after me, especially in medicine.

Many of my medical teams were composed mostly of young people - high school students, college students, and postgraduate trainees, including physicians and nurses. I found it incredibly rewarding to work alongside so many younger team members. More significantly, I realized they yearned for mentorship, encouragement, education, and investment in their growth. Although they might not explicitly say this, I learned to understand the unique "silent" language each of them used to convey this need.

In 2014, I was offered the opportunity to become a senior leader in a physician executive role with the nearby health system. Initially, I was a bit skeptical. In fact, I threw the application in the trash in my office. Then I had an epiphany! As I thought about the medical staff, for which I would be responsible, I realized that the majority of the physicians were anywhere from 10 to over 30 years younger than me! In other words, they were the ones I wanted to invest in, teach, encourage, and mentor! With a little push from a few key people, I accepted the position. As the Vice President of Medical Affairs, I faced numerous challenges, but the one that troubled me the most was the provider burnout, a critical issue of epidemic proportions. I know burnout, having gone through it myself. It was a terrible time. Emotional pain is the worst pain. Too often, it leads to despair and its brother, hopelessness. To live without hope is merely to exist, not truly to live.

I kept thinking about what I could do to better support and help the medical staff. They needed encouragement, to know that someone cared about them, appreciated them, and valued them. I decided to write stories, which I called "Bugle Notes" (this name dates back to my earliest days at West Point), about things I have experienced that would be motivational for them. Initially, I wrote one story a month. After the first 3 months, I had received no feedback from the medical staff, but I chose to continue writing to them. One day, I got an email from a doctor expressing gratitude for the "Bugle Notes" and asking me to continue writing them! More emails soon followed, and people started approaching me in the hospital, sharing how my previous story affected them and thanking me. With time, I began writing two stories each month and continued doing so for the rest of my tenure as VPMA.

My initial plan was to compile these "Bugle Notes" into a book for my three sons: Chris, Vaughan, and David. In many ways, these are the stories of my life, and I wanted them to have them. Unexpectedly, I had many people encourage me to publish them!

To all those who read even one of them, I sincerely thank you. They come directly from my heart.

Andy Lamb, MD 2025

SECTION I
ON BEING
HUMAN

CHAPTER 1

Final Words

I cared for the couple for 20 years. Both of them are in their 80s; she is a retired nurse, and he runs a business. They were so typical of the "greatest generation": tough, resilient, hard-working, deeply faithful, and fervently independent - those characteristics that enabled them to survive the Great Depression, World War II, and all the many challenges that come with life. They have experienced a good deal of joy, but have also endured significant pain, particularly the sudden loss of a child.

Now, in their waning old age, they were facing their greatest challenge, and I was intimately involved with them. They were dying; she of Alzheimer's, and he of severe pulmonary fibrosis; each one's life slowly diminishing in a way unique to their condition.

It was hard, very hard, to watch this unfold, though I have been here too many times with other patients during my 28-plus years as an Internal Medicine Specialist.

Caring for those going through the dying process is always a difficult and emotionally draining task. Over time, many experiences become a blur, and memories fade. But occasionally, a special person—or, in this case, a couple—enters your life, and their existence, along with everything it includes, becomes deeply intertwined with yours. There is often a final event, as well, that is etched forever in your mind and touches your soul. That event occurred last week. It moved me to tears, yet strangely enough, it also brought joy.

He was in with a care provider from his new home, where he and his wife had just moved, an assisted living facility with an Alzheimer's unit. He was no longer able to care for her as his lung disease and increasingly frequent hospital admissions were taking an irreversible toll on his body and remaining strength. He required oxygen continuously, and this once-strong man could now only walk 15-20 feet before having to stop and catch his breath. So, he made the decision to break away from their home of 60 years and move into a new "home". He did not want anyone else to make this decision on his behalf. It was the one thing he could do that would also ensure his wife would be cared for, even though she did not understand why this was happening. It was hard, terribly hard. In their new home, she was not able to stay with him. Her increasing agitation, combativeness, and paranoia precluded this. She had to remain in the "unit". Being a physician, I understand that Alzheimer's does far more than just take away one's memory.

I had not seen him in several months. Fortunately, he had not had a repeated visit to the hospital, and he was deemed "stable", a good word in medicine. However, he was noticeably thinner and weaker. There was gloom in his voice, his eyes, and his demeanor that I had not seen previously. We discussed his health issues and whether there was anything else we could do. By any clinical standard, he was depressed, and I had already addressed this. All I could see, though, were the tears brimming in his eyes and the trembling in his voice. All I could feel was the profound sadness permeating the room as he told me how difficult this move had been, and how hard it was to see "the love of his life" in such a state. What can one do or say in such scenarios? I did the only thing I could think of. I took his hands in mine, hands tough and calloused, that had done and felt so much in a lifetime, and I prayed with him. This was not the first time that we had done this. It was our practice through the years. As we finished, tears streaming down his face, his lips trembling with emotion, he said these final words: "I love you." He slowly got to his feet, embraced me, and walked away. As I observed him painfully making his way down the hall with a walker and oxygen by his side, tears welled up in my eyes— tears of both sadness and sorrow. Suddenly, I found myself grateful that I was in a profession that allowed me the privilege of being intimately involved in the lives of people, both the good and the bad, the joyful and the sad. When all has been done medically, then the real "art of medicine" begins: the warmth of love given through a touch and the speaking of words like "I love you" - the final words that are a precious reminder of why I went into medicine.

"I love you, too."

CHAPTER 2

A Terrible Time

His breathing was rapid and shallow; Oxygen in place, his eyes stared at the ceiling of the hospital room. He was a soldier in his late 20s, his once strong body now emaciated, a shell of its former self. His arms rested on top of the bedsheet, bluish nodular lesions of Kaposi's sarcoma landscaping them as they did the rest of his body. His lungs appeared as a "white-out" on the X-ray due to the relentless spread of the unusual cancer. It was 1985. He was dying of AIDS. They all died, all of them, from this frightening and poorly understood disease. It was a terrible time.

I was in my Internal Medicine residency at Eisenhower Army Medical Center at Fort Gordon, Georgia, outside of Augusta. The AIDS epidemic was exploding, and the military was not immune. Eisenhower was the HIV referral center for all the Armed Forces, their families, and retirees for the Southeastern US, Europe, and Panama. By the end of my first year of training, I was caring for a medicine floor of twenty or more soldiers in varying stages of HIV/AIDS.

I was halfway through what was to be a 15-month stretch of inpatient care without a day off. Each week, a 100-hour-plus marathon of unceasing work intermixed with a call every fortnight, 36 to 40 hours of punishing sleeplessness. I was thankful it was only every 4th night. My mind and body were in "survival mode", my own humanity replaced by a depersonalized, robotic self that I did not recognize. Patients were no longer people to me; they were work; more work in a limitless sea of diseases and death in which I frantically tread.

Fear, prejudice, and ignorance permeated the culture of the time. People were afraid to be in the same room with an infected individual, especially those in the last stages of the disease. Sons, husbands, and fathers, at times, were abandoned by those they loved, never to see them again. They were all gay, these young men in the prime of their lives. They had simply kept it hidden from a society that could not accept who they were. Their identity became equivalent to the virus; shame, embarrassment, and guilt further drove their families away from them. No one came to see him with caring words or the warmth of love given through a human touch. The only people to do so were the doctors and nurses. We battled our own fears and prejudices, only to have them slowly eroded as our hearts were broken by what we witnessed. No longer did I see him as just "more work". Finally, I started seeing him as a human being in need of acknowledgement, affirmation, non-judgmental condolence, and, most of all, a touch given with compassion, care, and love. No one should experience what he was going through, no matter who they were, what they did, or what they believed. He deserved the same dignity we all do. The protective wall I had built around me came crumbling down, and my heart emerged again. The nurses and I loved on him until his breath became air. He was not alone.

It was a terrible time, a sad time. It was a time that changed me as a person, and I am forever grateful for such humbling experiences. I will always remember that young man from so long ago. He gave me back my humanity. Now, HIV is a chronic, treatable disease, but in the beginning....

Thank you for your heart of compassion, empathy, and caring.

CHAPTER 3

They Are Not Alone

Several years ago, I watched an interview featuring nurses who attended to a man succumbing to Ebola. Their words and actions continue to ring true today, during the ongoing COVID-19 pandemic, as they did then.

I was deeply moved by their compassion for this man dying a horrible death. They did all they could for him, not only out of a sense of duty, but also emotionally, with all their heart and compassion. They spoke of the fear that had gripped them due to the personal risks they faced. Yet, each voluntarily chose to care for him. When asked why they would put their lives at risk, they did not give the answer you would expect - I am a nurse, this is what I am trained to do; I'm a professional; but the answer that they gave moved me to tears, "He was alone because his family could not be with him." Each of these nurses did not want him to be alone, to die with no one to love him, comfort him, or care for him. They described how, despite wearing all the protective gear, they would hold his hand, speak words of comfort and reassurance, and toward the end, simply hold him. The nurse caring for him on his deathbed said that tears were coming down the patient's face after being placed on the ventilator. She tried to reassure him that everything would be okay, but 15 minutes later, he died. The nurse cried and said," It was the worst day of my life."

Each of these amazing nurses risked their lives to care for a man they did not know. Sure, part of the reason was that it was their job; they were trained to do this. But as you listened to their words, the emotion in their voice, saw the trembling of their chin, and the tears flowing from their eyes, there was a much bigger reason. They truly had compassion for this man, and since he was alone and his family could not be with him, they became his surrogate family. They lovingly cared for him, washed his face with a cold wash rag, dealt with the copious diarrhea and vomiting, changed his clothing and linen, and administered his medications and fluids despite the risk to themselves. More importantly, though, they simply loved him with their kind words and actions.

When medical treatment fails and nothing else can be done, then the real "art of medicine" begins - the art of compassion, caring, and love, wiping away tears, speaking words of comfort, and simply holding them.

Watching these interviews on TV took me back to the earliest days of my internal medicine training during the 1980s. I trained at the peak of the AIDS epidemic before any adequate treatment was available. I cared for scores of young men with HIV or dying of AIDS. I was present with them until their last breaths. This was a time, much like with the Ebola scares, where there was much fear, uncertainty, and sadly, prejudice. As a result, we, the nurses and house staff, watched repeatedly as these young men were abandoned by their families - parents, wives, siblings, and friends out of fear and ignorance. As a result, they were also alone. I will never forget how dramatically that impacted me. No one deserves to be abandoned like that, no one should be left to suffer and die alone. We gave them the best treatment possible, very much aware of their fate. When nothing more could be done, we sat with them, held their hand, comforted them, and let them know we cared, that they were not alone.

Is this not what medicine should be about? Is this not why we entered this field? There's so much more to medicine than simply the medical and surgical treatment side, as important as that is. There's the human side - the compassion, caring, and loving warmth of a human touch; the knowing that at a patient's time of greatest fear, helplessness, and need, they are not alone, we are there for them.

Medicine is hard, very hard. There are times when we need to be reminded why we went into this profession, this calling, lest we forget in the busyness of our days with all the many demands placed upon us. At times, it's important to reflect on the last time we were there, so they would not be alone. Thank you for the sacrifices you make each and every day for your patients, community, and families. You are not alone in this journey.

CHAPTER 4

Stained-Glass Windows

I recently saw a powerful video about an amazing nurse who was a foster mother to children dying of cancer. She lovingly cared for them no matter the circumstance, the difficulties, or the heartbreak that came with each and every death of one of these precious children. It broke my heart to see and hear her story. It caused me to reflect on how fortunate we are in healthcare to have people with hearts much like hers, physicians and nurses alike. It was a special reminder of what a unique and privileged opportunity we have to care for those in the last days or weeks of their life. This time can be heartbreaking, but it can be soul-healing as well.

When asked how she could continue to love and care for these children, all of whom die, she said one of the most moving things I have ever heard:

"We invest deeply and we ache terribly when these kids die, but our hearts are like stained-glass windows. These windows are made of broken glass which has been forged back together, and those windows are even stronger and more beautiful for having been broken."

Hearts like "stained-glass windows", made of broken glass, forged back together, only to be even stronger and more beautiful for having been broken! Does this not speak to the essence of why we do what we do, but also the price we pay as nurses and physicians, as human beings, for being willing to do so? Nurses understand this because they are the ones who spend the most time caring for patients and addressing their needs, regardless of the challenges involved. Physicians understand because they have the ultimate responsibility for every patient and bear the burden that goes with that responsibility.

To all the physicians, advanced practice providers, and nurses, I say thank you. Thank you for having hearts that, with time, have become more and more like "stained-glass windows", broken all too often only to be forged back together, stronger and more exquisite. You are the "heart" of medicine. You selflessly and tirelessly care for those who are sick and suffering, and afraid and alone, and frightened. In their time of greatest need, you are their hope-giver. But when all else fails, you do the only thing left to do: you give a part of yourself, but at the cost of this "stained-glass window". It is a heavy price to pay, but you are stronger and more beautiful for having done so. Thank you for the many sacrifices you make every day, and thank you for the difference you make in every patient's life.

CHAPTER 5

When All Else Fails

During my 30 years in medicine, and especially as I began leading medical missions in 2005 to the poorest countries in the world, I have seen significant need and tragedy, along with heartbreak. Altogether, it becomes overwhelming, and despite our best medical efforts to help, we often fail. What do you do when all else fails? What do you do when someone has lost all hope and you feel you have nothing else to offer?

In his book "Unspeakable: Facing Up to the Challenge of Evil", the noted author and speaker Os Guinness recounts a powerfully moving story of harboring incredible faith in the face of unimaginable horror. He tells of Baroness Caroline Cox, who is known as the "Mother Teresa of the war-torn poor". To countless individuals in need around the globe, she embodies "love in action" and serves as a strong advocate for the overlooked. Regardless of the color, creed, or race of the victims of war - those who have been maimed and raped, their families robbed, killed, or taken into slavery - she reaches out with food, clothes, and medicine. Often when she arrives, the people greet her with the words: "Thank God you've come. We thought the world had forgotten us."

She was once asked to retell both her worst and best moments during all her journeys of mercy and compassion. "The worst?" She thought for a moment, then described with brutal simplicity what it was like to enter a Dinka village after Sudanese government-backed soldiers had left:

"The stench of death was overpowering. More than a hundred corpses lay where they had been savagely butchered. Men, women, children, even cattle, had been cut down or herded into captivity to be carried north as slaves. Straw huts were ablaze, crops had been razed, and devastation and death confronted the eyes everywhere. Worst of all was the knowledge that the militia would return with their gunships and Kalashnikov rifles, and the area's villages would once again lie naked before the ferocity and bloodlust of their attackers from the North. Genocide is an overworked word and one I never use without meaning it. But I mean it."

And the best moment? It came right after the worst. With the raiders gone and the results of their cruelty all around, the few women still alive - husbands slain, children kidnapped into slavery, homes ruined and they themselves brutally raped- were all pulling themselves together. Their first instinctive act was to make tiny crosses out of sticks lying on the ground and to push them into the earth. What were they doing? One might guess that they were fashioning instant memorials to those they had lost. No, the crudely formed crossed sticks, pressed into the ground at the moment when their bodies reeled and their hearts bled, were the emblems of their faith. They served a God who they believed knew pain as they knew pain. Blinded by pain and grief themselves, horribly aware that the world would neither know nor care about their plight, they still staked their lives on the conviction that there was One who knew and cared."

"They were not alone."

Hopefully, none of us will ever face such horror. But what each of you faces each day are patients and families who often are going through an illness or personal tragedy that, at the time, is truly overwhelming for them, just as devastating, just as heartbreaking, just as life-changing. And when faced with these patients and their families, sometimes even our best medical efforts fail.

Sometimes, even our best attempts to give hope and be "hope-givers" are not enough. What do you do then? Medical training does not teach what to do when there is nothing left medically to do and all hope seems gone, at least I wasn't. This is when, I believe, there is only one thing left to do - to give what I call "the warmth of love" that comes through a loving touch, holding a hand, giving a hug, and more powerfully, shedding tears as you share their pain, hurt, and hopelessness. Have you ever done this with someone? It is a frightening thing to be so transparent. This is especially true for those in healthcare who have learned to compartmentalize their emotions. I believe, and I have experienced this many times, that the true "art of medicine", the human side of medicine, comes through brightest and most powerfully at such moments when we allow ourselves to be their "tears". Are you willing to be "tears" for your patients and their families? If you are, you will find a renewed joy as you experience real medicine once again, and your patients will know that they are not alone.

As always, thank you for the hard, selfless, and caring work you do every day.

CHAPTER 6

The Question

"Will I ever get better, Andrew?" my mother asked me while she lay in bed, too feeble to sit up, unable to eat, her myelofibrosis in the final stages of its relentless course. Her question stunned me – did she not know she was dying? How could she not? Was she in complete denial? Was she simply grasping for a final chance at hope when all seemed hopeless? Reality quickly set in. She did not know or at least fully comprehend that she was dying, despite the countless doctor's visits, multiple hospitalizations, surgeries, failed treatments, and unrelenting blood transfusions.

The answer was all too simple to me: poor communication. Throughout the nearly year-long course of her aggressive disease, her Hematologist had not taken the time to speak truth to her nor to the rest of my family. She was "too busy" to return calls or take the time in her office to address their growing concerns and fears.

With each round of hospitalization and failed treatment, frustration and anger grew.

I became my mother's doctor in the sense that my family sought me for unresolved questions and decisions that needed to be made. I was no longer her son, which was all I wanted to be. I did not want to be her doctor. I only wanted to be her son and love her through this difficult fate. But the questions arose, decisions had to be made, and my family needed help. It was a terrible time, and it only became worse as time passed.

I began taking weekly trips to Alabama from my home in North Carolina, leaving Friday at noon and returning late Sunday, a seven hour drive each way, so I could see her, support my family, and address the issues that inevitably emerged. This went on for 6 months, missing only the weekends when I was on call. My full-time private practice continued, as did the hospital calls (before the advent of Hospitalists). In addition, I was the President of a multi-specialty clinic, and I had a rebellious teenager. These only added to the adversity.

Then one weekend, as I sat on the edge of her bed, she asked the question. With a quivering voice and welled-up eyes, I told her the truth, "No, Mama, you won't get better." I could not bring myself to tell her she would most likely die in a few days. She looked at me, rolled on her side, closed her eyes, and said her final words to me, "I love you, Andrew."

I was angry. Angry at the world. Angry that I had to be the one to speak those words to her. Angry that I could not be just her son. Angry at that poor excuse of a physician who couldn't take the time to speak words of truth, support, and comfort to my mother and family. I went upstairs to my room, closed the door, and cried. I cried in anger, frustration, and grief, and for the lost opportunity to simply be her son. My sister came to the room and we held each other, and I cried even more. My mother died 2 days later at the age of 66.

Have you ever had to take on the role of a physician within your family? If so, were you equally surprised? Our families love us, they trust us, and we understand the language of medicine. The physician side of us wants to help, to make things better, and to prevent their suffering. Being a physician is hard enough without having to take on this heavy responsibility. There comes a time when a health crisis hits our family. At this crucial time, we should be able to be the son, the daughter, the husband, the wife, the mother, the father, and not the physician. My mother needed her son, her little boy, not her son, the doctor. I should have drawn a line in the sand, but I did not. If and when your turn comes, draw that line, make that boundary, and do your best not to cross it.

I grieve the missed opportunity to have simply loved her as a son in her final days. I tried to do that, but circumstances prevented me from doing so. Don't let that happen to you. And don't become the physician who sees medicine only as a job, instead of a true calling —a profession where compassion, caring, and relationships make a difference in the lives of patients and their families. My mother deserved such a physician.

CHAPTER 7

The Best of Their Generation

In Ken Burns's epic documentary on the Vietnam War, one statement by a veteran caused me to pause and think. The veteran said, "Those who fought in World War II have been called the 'Greatest Generation'. I believe every war brings out the best of its generation." I realized he was right. The best of each generation has always responded in one way or another to the call of their country. They and their families did so at great personal cost and sacrifice.

Hearing those words made me think of all of you. Why? For similar reasons. At great personal costs and sacrifice, each of you has trained and prepared for your own "war" as you battle every day for those who have entrusted their care, and often their lives, to you. Whether you trained 30 or more years ago, as I did, or just finished, you represent "the best of your generation". Every year, medicine becomes increasingly challenging and demands greater sacrifices. Patients are older, sicker, and more complicated. Yet medically and technologically, there is far more we can do for them. Unrealistic expectations from patients and their families, the rising costs of healthcare, the increasing administrative burdens, especially those associated with electronic medical records (EMR), and the continuing loss of autonomy have created an environment that is arguably the most challenging for physicians.

I write this "Bugle Notes" to acknowledge that you are the best of your generation. I am humbled and honored to serve you and, in many cases, to have worked alongside you in the care of our patients. Please accept my deepest gratitude for your sacrifice and the sacrifice of your families. Thank you for your willingness to answer the call to care for those in need. Finally, thank you for always striving to provide the best care possible to our patients and our community.

Postscript- I wrote this "Bugle Notes" in 2017. We are now in a war against a terrible, invisible foe, COVID-19. "The best of their generation" are at the front lines fighting right now. We all owe them a tremendous depth of gratitude and applause as they sacrifice much for us all.

CHAPTER 8

A Silent Epidemic

She reached for my hand, her hands wrinkled and gnarled; the skin fragile, translucent, road-mapped by bluish veins; hands that had done much in her 87 years of living. She looked at me from her hospital bed and, with her voice trembling, her eyes tearing, spoke the words that pierced my heart - "Can I stay here? Everyone is so kind. I am all alone now. I have no family, no friends left. I have no one to talk to. Please let me stay."

Her severe lung disease was taking a toll on her physical and mental health, as the inevitable downward spiral continued. Despite this, she remained fiercely independent, tough, and resilient, so typical of her generation. Her tough exterior, though, was crumbling, and along with it, her strength and will, too. She gripped my hand a little tighter, and her eyes pleaded. The loneliness that now defined her life had become unbearable. Its unwelcome companions, despair and hopelessness, now resident in her heart, replaced any remaining hope and joy. Without hope, she no longer lived life; she only existed, day by day. I reassured her that she would receive all the support and help she needed at home. With that, she asked me to pray for her. I did so, and when I finished, she prayed for me as well—a precious reminder of the sacredness of the doctor-patient relationship. She gave a nod of resignation, released my hand, and looked away. I begrudgingly placed the order to discharge her.

Her loneliness had become personal to me, and in doing so, it had become an integral part of my reality. How many times had I missed the silent cries of others; cries from the depths of their loneliness and isolation; cries for acknowledgment, affirmation, for someone to hear "their story" and, in doing so, validate who they were as human beings? How many patients needed more than physical healing? How many simply needed the warmth of love given through a human touch or words spoken with kindness and empathy? How many of them never expressed their silent wishes to me, and I remained equally oblivious?

Loneliness is a silent epidemic crying out to be heard. More patients to be seen, beds to free up, documentation to complete, clicks on the EMR to make, families to talk to - the list goes on, all smothering the cry. We build walls, wear masks, and put on blinders to protect ourselves from the pain, suffering, and heartbreak inherent to medicine. In doing so, we can lose sight of the person in front of us and the humanness of that person. Relationships are an intimate human need; the absence of which creates an internal void that needs to be filled. Loneliness, with its despair and hopelessness, waits to do that.

May we recognize the loneliness that envelopes so many. Even if words are not spoken, the message is still received - notice me, see me; I am alone, and I need that warmth of love....

CHAPTER 9

Woman by the Elevator

"How long have you been married?" The question came from a young woman kneeling down by the elevator in the hotel where my wife and I were staying while in Seattle. We were there to celebrate our 40th wedding anniversary with an Alaskan cruise. I hadn't even noticed her as my wife and I were busy talking about the day. She appeared to be in her twenties. Her appearance was that of a person seeking attention, characterized by excessive makeup and provocative clothing. Maybe she was masking something deeper? She held a hotel key in her left hand as she tried to frantically shove a pair of jeans and a T-shirt into a small bag. Her purpose for the evening seemed apparent. It was her unsolicited question and the words that followed that surprised my wife and me, and later came to haunt us.

I answered, "We have been married for 40 years, and in fact, we are here to celebrate our anniversary." As she continued stuffing the clothes into the bag, she looked up and said, "Just be thankful you aren't a Millennial." We were both stunned by this comment and did not know what to say. She then said, "My parents were married for 12 years. Stay married." She returned to packing her bag without saying another word. The elevator door opened, and my wife and I got in. However, she stayed kneeling, intent on finishing the packing. I had the distinct impression she was purposefully delaying an inevitable event.

In the elevator, my wife and I looked at each other, trying to make sense of what had just happened. We considered going back to find her. There had been such sadness in her voice and on her face. Was she involved in human trafficking? Was she a runaway trying to survive the best she could? What was the "story" behind those words? Even now, two weeks later, we think about her, and the words she said, words that were more like those of a sad little girl instead of a young woman. We remain haunted by that brief encounter. We should have done something for her, yet we did not. Why? We both have compassion and concern for others, yet we did nothing. What will happen to her? We will never know. We only know we missed an opportunity to help someone who cried out to us for help.

I wonder how many times in the 30 years of my practice did I miss the subtle cries for help from my own patients because I was too busy to "hear" them. We live in a hurting world. It is easy to overlook the hurt, pain, and hopelessness around us because of the hustle of our own lives or perhaps even our own personal struggles and difficulties. My hope is that each of us will hear that cry for help, however subtle it may be, and take action. We are in a unique position to make a genuine difference in the lives of people in more ways than just medically. We only need to be willing to listen for that cry. Thank you for living a life that makes a difference to others every day.

CHAPTER 10

Every Tear Earned

Have you ever found yourself in front of a patient, not knowing what to say or do? Maybe you just told them they had cancer, or that the last treatment option had failed, or that a loved one had died. I have, many times, and I always felt helpless, inept, and alone while doubting my abilities as a physician. Medical school had not prepared me for this. I learned firsthand, one difficult and sometimes heartbreaking experience after another. I came to understand that often, in those moments, patients do not need another person talking to them. They need someone with them. Words will go unheard as they are already overwhelmed trying to process what has happened. Instead, I sat and I listened.

I held their hand. Sometimes we prayed.

Have you ever cried with a patient? I was taught that men don't cry, and by extension, that applied to boys as well. Early in my life, I struggled with this, though in an innocent way. Movies or books that moved me were a real challenge! "Shenandoah" or the classic movie "Old Yeller" did me in! But worst of all was the book, "Where the Red Fern Grows", the classic tear-jerker of all time, especially when your 6th-grade teacher was cruel enough to read it out loud to the class! It was torture. Despite my best attempts, the tears would come. As nonchalantly as possible, I would wipe away the tears, pretending to be scratching an itch. I dared not look at another person. It was the same for all the boys, even the class bully. The girls, of course, cried openly without a shred of shame. Girls were allowed to cry, and boys were not. It wasn't fair.

Here I am speaking of different tears, though. Not the tears of a Romantic or of an innocent child. Instead, the tears "earned" through years of intense training, hard work, sacrifice, giving of yourself to patients, and grieving, often silently, when they died. The "sacred trust" that exists between providers and patients creates a bond and intimacy unlike any other profession. You learn to compartmentalize your emotions. Otherwise, you could not continue. It would become too much. It is already too much for many.

When all else has failed and there is nothing medically left to do, then the real "Art of Medicine" can happen through the warmth of a human touch, a comforting hug, and the sharing of tears, where every tear is earned. Through these tears, a healing of the heart can happen.

CHAPTER 11

Words of Comfort

Abraham Verghese's must read book, "Cutting for Stone," compellingly explores the human aspect of medicine. It is a poignant reminder of the sanctity within medicine created by the unique bond that is the doctor-patient relationship; a relationship, I believe, in peril. We are allowed into that most intimate space, an individual's life during their most vulnerable and fearful moments.

In the book, a prominent surgeon reads a letter to the house staff from a grieving mother. Her words are piercing and convicting.

"... I cannot get over one image, a last image that could have been different. I saw that my son was terrified, and there was no one there to address his fears. Everyone ignored him. The doctors were busy with his body. They cared only about his chest and belly, not about the little boy who was in fear. Yes, he was a man, but at such a vulnerable moment, he was reduced to a little boy. I saw no sign of the slightest bit of human kindness. My son's last conscious memory will be of people ignoring him. My last memory of him will be of my little boy watching in terror as his mother is escorted out of the room. It is the graven image I will carry it to my own deathbed. The fact that people were attentive to his body does not compensate for their ignoring his being."

Utter silence followed. He then asks, "What treatment in an emergency is administered by ear?" The answer - "words of comfort". I was struck by the simplicity of the answer and yet the depth of its meaning. Memories of previous patients surfaced from the recesses of my mind. Did I give them "words of comfort" they desperately needed, or was I too focused on the tasks at hand, the myriad things that had to be done?

Doctors are trained exceptionally well medically and surgically. How well, though, are we prepared to give "words of comfort"? I want to think I always spoke these words to my patients, but did I? I believe I did. I hope I did. How tragic to not receive this most basic act of humaneness; to be reduced instead to an existence personified by high-tech monitors, tubing, IV drips; their world a cacophony of sights and sounds; no longer seen as a person, a human being with dignity, a mother's "little boy or girl".

There will always be the human side to medicine. It is predicated on relationships intentionally offered, developed, and nurtured. Without this personal connection, we chance ignoring their "being", and who they are as a person of worth, deserving of kindness and compassion.

Through medical missions, I learned that the needs of others do not become real to us until they become personal. They become personal when we experience them through the warmth of love given through a touch, acts of kindness and service, or words of hope and comfort. Without these, Verghese quotes, "Call no man happy until he dies."

We fail our patients when we forget the power that words of kindness and acts of comfort carry. May we always remember this simple "treatment" and, in doing so, remember from whence we first loved medicine.

CHAPTER 12

The Accident

It was a beautiful spring day. My wife and I were returning from UNC-Chapel Hill after visiting our oldest son. Driving on Highway 54, I suddenly saw a young woman on the left side of the road frantically waving her arms and screaming.

Behind her, a pickup truck had crashed into a tree. I immediately stopped the car. That's when I saw him. Lying, unmoving, and on his back was a young man in his 20s. I quickly got out of the car and ran to him. He had significant head trauma. There was a large, gaping, right parietal skull fracture. His brain exposed. He was bleeding from his nose, mouth, and ears. Surprisingly, he was breathing and had a pulse. A few feet away, his girlfriend screamed hysterically as my wife tried to calm her.

A woman appeared on the opposite side of him, quickly saying she was a nurse. At that moment, he stopped breathing, and what was real suddenly became surreal. What do I do? Do I start CPR knowing I would expose myself to his blood and the potential risks that come with it? Do I do nothing and let him die? And what about his distraught girlfriend standing over me? Memories of the scores of HIV infected soldiers I cared for in the Army during the mid-1980s came flooding back to me. All died horrible deaths from AIDS. My attention returned to the havoc in front of me.

I had to make a decision. Everyone was waiting - the young woman, the unknown nurse, my wife, and now several newly arrived bystanders - all waiting to see what I would do.

I gave him two breaths. The nurse started chest compressions. With each breath, my blood exposure increased, yet I continued. Why? That question came later.

Later, after the EMS arrived and took over, after a kind woman took me to her home to clean off the blood, after I returned to the site, the man, the girlfriend, the ambulance no longer there; after the surreal became real again. Did this really happen? My thoughts returned to those soldiers....

From my car, I called the ED at the hospital where I worked. I relayed what had happened to the ED physician, a good friend. He was waiting for the patient to arrive as EMS had called with their report. He told me they would do all they could. He quickly added that he would get the necessary blood tests and call me as soon as they returned. As I waited for his call, my thoughts went back to my family. Any fear or anxiety for myself was replaced by fear of what this could mean to my family should I become infected.

Did I make the right choice? Do a patient's needs take precedence over our families and ourselves? My years of education, training, and experience affirm yes. But what would my family think? My wife was present, yet I did not ask her opinion; I simply acted. I believe I made the right decision. I would never fault anyone for making a different one.

The call came. He died. His HIV was negative, as were subsequently all the other tests. The next day, I bought a portable CPR mask to keep in my car at all times.

CHAPTER 13

If They Only Knew

I recently read a story that struck close to home for me, and I suspect for nearly all of you at one time or another in your medical careers. It was a story of a surgeon who was called in urgently to the ED for a seriously injured young boy. The surgeon arrived as soon as he could, only to be confronted by an irate father for being late and accusing the surgeon of being uncaring, self-centered, and money-driven. It was an ugly scene. The surgeon remained calm, apologized, and told the father he would do all he could to help his son. Even this did not appease the father and he continued to verbally harangue the surgeon. After the surgery, the surgeon spoke to the father, explained that all went well and full recovery was expected. He then promptly left. The man told the OR nurse that he couldn't believe how callous and cold the surgeon was, first for being late, and second for being so brusque with his departure after the surgery. The nurse then told him "The rest of the story".

The surgeon arrived late because his son had died in an accident just days earlier. He was attending his son's funeral when he received a call back to the emergency department. The nurse informed the father, "He left his own son's funeral so he could take care of your son." Unsurprisingly, the man had nothing more to say.

Most of us have been in similar situations. I can think of times, maybe not as tragic as this, but still difficult times, when I was running behind only to be confronted by an angry patient or family member for being so thoughtless and uncaring as to waste their time. If they only knew....

The reason I was late seeing you, even though you were the first patient of the day, was that I had just left the ICU, where a patient whom I had cared for through the years had died. I spent over 45 minutes with the grieving family.

I have been in the hospital on call for over 24 hours, working all night, rounding since six in the morning, only to have the son of a newly admitted, unassigned patient, come in from out of town, irate that no one had called him. Notably, this son had not seen his mother in several years.

The patient I saw before you was sobbing when I walked into the exam room to see her for what should have been a routine 15-minute appointment. She had just found out her husband of 20 years was having an affair and wanted a divorce. She was devastated. It took longer than 15 minutes to see her.

Only minutes earlier, I told a patient of 20 years and his family that he has Alzheimer's. How do you do that in 15 minutes?

The previous patient was a nurse with whom I had worked for many years. She was in to review test results. The test showed metastatic cancer throughout her liver. She was 46 with a husband and 3 children at home.

My own mother in Alabama is dying. Her doctor isn't communicating with my father, brothers, and sister. They are turning to me for answers. I am personally burned out, and it's all I can do to see one more patient. It's all I can do to make it through each day. It is all I could do to remain in the room because I simply didn't care anymore.

You have your own "if they only knew" stories, I am sure. Medicine is challenging, and it is becoming even more so. Patients and their families are becoming increasingly demanding, with expectations that are often unrealistic. They want you to treat them as if they are the most important person in your life. They expect you to always be smiling, happy, and engaging. You try to do that, but sometimes, despite your best efforts, you simply can't because "if they only knew…"

You're not alone in this hard work that is medicine. There are people who care about you. I am one of them. I know how hard it can be.

Thank you for persevering, even when you feel you can no longer continue. You are valued. You are appreciated. You are making a difference every day in the lives of others.

CHAPTER 14

Betsy

I will never forget the moment I heard the news. "What! No way! You are joking, right?" But she wasn't. "No, Andy, Betsy was just diagnosed with Stage IV colon cancer."

I was shocked. How could it be? Betsy was only 32 years old. She had finally met the man of her dreams after years of wondering if she ever would. They had been married for only three months! This could not be happening. This is Betsy, the young, energetic, loving, caring, and smiling nurse with whom I have served on many medical missions. She was healthy! She had no risk factors - no Inflammatory Bowel Disease, no family history. The reality finally began to set in — chances were she would not live another 1-2 years.

She was determined to beat this, and thus began what has been a one and a half year battle that continues to this day. Unfortunately, it is a battle she was losing, and she knew it. Yet, she has continued to fight heroically, with the loving support of her husband, as she has sought out the latest treatment options. She has tried every experimental protocol for which she qualified. Some have slowed the disease briefly, but most have only caused severe, incapacitating side effects.

I maintain close communication with Betsy, particularly through the "Caring Bridge" website. She regularly shares updates on her physical condition while also candidly discussing her emotional and spiritual challenges. My heart breaks for her as she increasingly writes about the harsh reality of her impending death. A miracle from God aside, she understands she has very little time left (and she possesses a strong faith). She expresses the heartbreak, deep sadness, and overwhelming grief that resonate profoundly within her soul.

She grieves that she will not have a long, full life with her husband, the man for whom she had prayed and waited all those years. She grieves that she will never have children and she loves children. She is the best aunt ever to her nieces! She mourns that she will not get to see them grow to adulthood. Most of all, she grieves the loss of what could have been, should have been.

Amidst everything, her faith remains the bedrock upon which she lives. Consequently, her life serves as an inspiration to those fortunate enough to know her. She consistently reminds us of the beauty that envelops us daily; of the blessings of our lives; and that each day deserves to be treasured as the gift it is.

I remember the last time I saw her. Many months after her initial diagnosis, followed by multiple surgeries and intense, debilitating chemotherapy, a close friend and I flew up to visit Betsy and her husband. We longed to see her. We needed to see her. At that time, it was uncertain if she would live another 6 months. We did all we could to make it as special a weekend as possible - dinner at a fine restaurant, a comedy play, where I vividly remember her holding her husband's hand, laying her head on his shoulder, and actually laughing! We provided prayer, words of encouragement, and love. Most of all, we listened to her as she poured her heart out to us.

As I departed, we embraced and said, "I love you." When I turned to go, the storm door shut behind me. My final sight of Betsy was her smiling through the sunlit glass. As we waved goodbye, it dawned on me that this might be the last time I saw her. Tears filled my eyes. Life is too brief, and our relationships are too precious to let the chaos of work and daily life overshadow this truth. When you find yourself enduring a "horrible, terrible, no good, very bad day," remember there's still much for which to be grateful. Each day is an opportunity to bring healing and hope to those in need.

CHAPTER 15

"But Steps to Your Eternity"

"But Steps to Eternity"

"You that seek what life is in death,

Now find it air that once was breath,

New names unknown, old names gone:

Till time end, bodies, but souls none.

Reader! Then make time, while you be,

But steps to your eternity."

Baron Brooke Fulke Greville, "Caelica 83"

I cried that Sunday morning while sitting by my fire pit. It was all I could do to keep from sobbing as I read the final pages of "When Breath Becomes Air" by Paul Kalanithi, MD. I frequently had to pause mid-page to collect myself before I could keep reading.

At 36 years old, on the verge of completing ten years of training as a neurosurgeon and neuroscientist, Paul Kalanithi was diagnosed with stage IV lung cancer. "When Breath Becomes Air" narrates his journey from a medical student striving to define a virtuous and meaningful life, to a neurosurgeon delving into the complexities of human identity, and ultimately to a patient and new father facing his own mortality.

He died in March 2015 while working on this book, leaving behind a wife and an 8-month-old daughter. The tragedy of his premature death was heart-wrenching to read. However, the words he wrote in those final months of his life are an unforgettable, life-offering reflection on the challenge of facing death, but also on the sacred relationship between doctor and patient. In his dying, he had much to teach about life, offering powerful lessons that are all too easy to forget in the busyness of a physician's life.

In the book's early chapters, he reflects on the challenges he encountered during the arduous initial years in neurosurgery residency, where he recognized his desensitization to the suffering and death that became all too familiar. Paul was concerned about losing sight of the sacred bond between doctor and patient. He understood that his highest aspiration wasn't merely to save lives—everyone eventually dies—but rather to help patients and their families comprehend illness and death. He noted, "When there's no place for the scalpel, words are the surgeon's only tool." I resonate with this truth as I have witnessed significant suffering and death, not only throughout my medical career but also during the global medical missions I lead. In moments when all else fails—be it medical or surgical treatments, experimental approaches, or last-resort holistic therapies— what options remain? Our scalpel, our medical interventions become the words we choose and the way we express them. The appropriate words, delivered with care, compassion, and a gentle touch, can heal in unimaginable ways. Conversely, words spoken without this intention can inflict wounds as severe as the sharpest scalpel.

He believed doctors had a duty to learn "What made that particular patient's life worth living or, if not, to allow the peace of death. Such power required deep responsibility. Yet most lives are lived with passivity toward death." Reading those words reminded me of the final scene in the movie "Braveheart," where the protagonist, William Wallace, portrayed by Mel Gibson, knowing his execution was imminent, said, "All men die, but few men truly live."

Paul grappled with the idea of his own mortality as he sought to understand what made his life meaningful. Ultimately, it was his daughter who gave him a reason to fight for life. When his wife asked, "What are you afraid or sad about?" he replied, "Leaving you." He realized that having a child would bring happiness to their family, and he couldn't stand the thought of leaving his wife without children after his passing. His wife feared that saying goodbye to their child would intensify his dying experience. He responded, "Wouldn't it be wonderful if it did?" They both believed that life wasn't merely about evading suffering. Instead of succumbing to death, they chose to continue living, refusing to "miss the dance."

He realized that life is precious and that its worth doesn't come from money, status, titles, or possessions. He referred to these as vanities that are hardly significant: a pursuit of the wind. He recognized that we are all "but steps to your eternity," yet few of us pause from our hectic lives long enough to truly understand this.

We all need reminders of this truth. We have received a precious gift—the ability to impact others' lives and live a meaningful existence. We hold the great privilege inherent in the sacred trust between physician and patient. In our pursuit of what matters most, may we discover life instead of death, and breath instead of mere air, as we recall that we are "but steps to your eternity". What truly matters to you?

CHAPTER 16

On Death and Dying

Death is inevitable. How we die, though, we can and should have more control over. In this country, we are fortunate to have access to Palliative Care and Hospice programs. In my view, these professionals are "angels on earth." They empower our patients, friends, and loved ones to maintain that control while being cared for with compassion and dignity. I am so appreciative of the hard work they do. Yet, our healthcare system overall is not doing as well in this arena.

In today's aging, over-medicalized, technological environment with increasingly challenging patient/family expectations, the concept of dying with dignity has become too uncommon. The highest expenditure of costs on patient care occurs in the last two months of a person's life, and all too often for futile reasons. Atul Gwande's book, "On Being Mortal", provides great insight into the current state and the high costs, not only financially, but also emotionally, on every person involved.

During my 30 years as an Internal Medicine Specialist, I cared for more dying patients than I can remember. Some patients' deaths, though, you never forget because of the circumstances surrounding it and the impact it had on you personally.

I cared for her husband and her during my time in the Army years ago. She was dying of pulmonary fibrosis. A woman of strong faith, she had a loving, supportive family. Her wish was to die at home, surrounded by her family, with grace and dignity. I developed a very close relationship with both of them. They were wonderful people and had become my friends.

One evening, I got a call from her husband—she was on the verge of death, and could I come by to visit her? I drove to their home, where I met him and the three daughters who had flown in from different states to be with their mother. By the time I arrived, she had died. I remember standing at the bedside with the family as the husband prayed. Afterwards, he thanked me for the care I had provided her.

It was the youngest daughter's birthday, and they planned to celebrate with cake and champagne. Then, something truly remarkable occurred. The daughter poured a glass for each of us and invited us outside to the patio. The night sky was clear, and the stars shone brightly. She raised her glass to the sky and thanked God for her mother's life and the blessing she had been to her, the family, and countless others. We raised our glasses in a toast, blending tears of sadness with tears of joy as we celebrated her birthday. Their mother, my patient and my friend, had her wish fulfilled.

Moments like this serve as a poignant reminder of the privilege we have to be so intimately involved in the lives of our patients. It is a humbling experience during these sacred moments, made all the more so by the privilege and the relationships that result from it. What you do so well every day in the care of others is truly hard work. It is important work. Thank you for caring, serving, and loving so well.

CHAPTER 17

A Good Death

In today's increasingly technological, data-driven, depersonalized world of healthcare, I wonder if the concept of "a good death" is even possible.

The COVID-19 pandemic, in particular, has caused me to reflect on this. What does it look like? How do you define it? As I did, a patient came to mind. He was a retired minister in his 80s. I had cared for his wife as well until she passed away a few years earlier. He missed her terribly and longed to be with her again. He faced his own significant health problems, severe ischemic cardiomyopathy with a left ventricular ejection fraction of less than 10% and a 10 cm abdominal aortic aneurysm. Either condition could prove fatal, and he lived with the knowledge that he could die at any moment. Surgery was no longer an option. Despite this, he lived every day to the fullest, always filled with joy! We often discussed how his death would be. One thing was certain: he was at peace with it because he knew he would be with God and with his beloved wife!

I clearly remember receiving the page from the ED one early morning: "Reverend was just brought in by EMS. His AAA has ruptured but he is still alert and wants to see you." Rushing to the ED, I found him lying in bed, surprisingly alert and aware. He never expressed any pain. Standing by his side, holding his hand and looking into his eyes, I noticed a calmness and peace that was unlike anything I had encountered before. He mentioned that he wasn't afraid; rather, he felt ready to see his God and his beloved wife. As his blood pressure continued to decline, he expressed his gratitude for my years of care and for my "listening heart." With tears, we prayed together, and just minutes after we finished, he lost consciousness and passed away peacefully.

It was "a good death". As I walked away, my mind trying to process what I had just experienced, I was reminded of how privileged I was to have been a part of this man's life and now his death and only because of the "sacred relationship" between a physician (or other providers as well) and a patient. We are allowed to enter into the most hallowed space of all - that moment between life and death, when "breath becomes air" and nothing else holds significance. May such moments remind you of the impact you have on your patients' lives. Your work is hard, but it is also sacred.

CHAPTER 18

The Hug

The cardiologist was urgently summoned to the emergency department for a 50-year-old man experiencing a heart attack. The patient suffered cardiac arrest eight times in the ED, but each time, he was successfully resuscitated. Eventually, he stabilized enough to be transferred to the cardiac lab. The cardiologist promptly spoke with the man's wife, explaining the plans and assuring her that they would do everything in their power to save her husband's life. As he was about to leave, he was deeply affected by the expression in her eyes. It conveyed not only fear, but also an overwhelming despair. He could sense that she believed she would never see her husband alive again.

The cardiac catheterization went well with stenting of the culprit lesion. Two hours later, this same man, who repeatedly evaded death only 3 hours before, was awake, sitting up, and eating in the ICU, completely alert and oriented with no neurological deficits!

When he saw her in the waiting room, her posture, her facial expressions, her overall demeanor, and, again, that look in her eyes, said, "He's dead. My husband is dead!" She braced herself to hear the words that would forever change her life. Instead, he gave her the news she least expected - he was going to make a complete recovery!

Then that unexpected moment arrived. She dashed toward him with arms outstretched and enveloped him in a joyful embrace, crying tears of happiness, and refused to let go! She clung to him while she continued to weep. It was a breathtaking moment captured in time. As she held him tightly, the cardiologist recalled thinking that this was the reason he pursued a career in medicine and that he truly made a difference! He walked away with a sense of contentment he had not felt in... how long?

"The hug," a familiar human gesture, can be life-giving and soul-nurturing when we find ourselves in "a valley of dry bones," longing for new breath. Such moments are rare, but when they occur, they stay with us forever

When was the last time you experienced a moment like this? When it does happen, do you appreciate it for the gift it is, a moment of joy, however brief?

There is still joy to be found in medicine. Look for it, embrace it, savor it because like "the hug", it will give you a glimpse into what could be again - joy in medicine. You deserve that, you need to have that again! Thanks for being there!

CHAPTER 19

Despair

I know how hard healthcare providers, especially physicians, work; the challenges they face; the obstacles they must overcome; the demands and stresses they endure every day as they do the hard work of medicine. It is not getting easier; it is only becoming more difficult, and healthcare providers are paying the price. We are resilient, though; our training has shaped us this way. We believe we can withstand any demand and do any job, no matter how overwhelming it may feel. But in the recesses of our minds, we know this isn't true, and for many reasons, we won't admit it. For me, it was the fear of being seen as weak, not good enough, and not having "what it takes." I was taught I could achieve anything and endure anything through my efforts alone - or so I believed.

Have you ever felt pain? I mean, real physical pain? Pain so unbearable it takes your breath away, you are afraid to move, and you can't stop the tears from flowing. I have, and the physical pain I felt was the worst I had ever known. It gave me a better understanding and deeper compassion for my patients who endure such pain. I could not imagine experiencing pain worse than what I had gone through. I was wrong.

There is a worse pain. Like me, others have experienced it. I know because I was at their side when they did. Too many are going through it right now and cannot endure it much longer. Like I was, they are on the precipice of a deep, dark pit called despair. Despair, with its brother hopelessness, is the worst pain of all. It is an emotional state that I still find difficult to put into words. But I know it. I have felt it. I have lived it and it is bad. Despair, at its worst, must be experienced to fully understand what I am describing. I hope no one else experiences it, but the reality is that most will experience it at some point in their life.

Have you ever experienced pain so visceral that it was hard to breathe? Have you ever been so overwhelmed with grief or heartbreak that you could not stop crying? Have you ever gone month after month with no joy, a complete loss of joy, to the point that you have forgotten what it feels like to have it? You cannot imagine ever feeling it again. Have you ever gone night after night unable to sleep because your mind is racing, you cannot stop your thoughts, and you lie there praying for sleep, but it doesn't come? Have you ever felt so hopeless that you couldn't imagine things ever getting better? Have you ever been at the bottom of a deep, dark pit and couldn't climb out? Have you ever felt so alone that no matter how loud or how long you cried out, no one heard you?

This is pain, and too many of our colleagues are experiencing it right now. You can label it however you like—depression, burnout, etc.—but these words fail to convey the depth of despair. You cope as best you can; sometimes you manage well, but more often, not so much. I know because I went through the same struggle. It was the hardest thing I've ever faced. What saved me and helped me escape this pit of despair? First and foremost, it was my faith in God. A significant second was finally opening up to a few friends, both medical and non-medical, whom I knew I could trust, with whom I felt safe, and who would love and support me.

How mistaken I was to try to do that alone because of pride, shame, embarrassment, or simply the fear of appearing weak! Trying to persevere through this alone is futile. Eventually, even your best coping strategies, greatest efforts, and strongest facades will falter, and the weight of despair will engulf you. Those you love and care about will endure that pain alongside you. Thankfully, there are individuals who genuinely care, willing to listen—whether they are professionally trained or, like me, who know what others are going through and are ready to assist in any way possible. You cannot face this journey alone. Too much is at stake. Medicine is challenging enough, and life can be even tougher without a support system. But there is hope. Life can be fulfilling again, and happiness can return! Despair doesn't have to dominate you. The pain can stop.

CHAPTER 20

"Breathless Expectation"

I recently read something in which the expression "breathless expectation" was used. It describes how a person should feel about not knowing what tomorrow may bring. This led me to think about the last time I experienced what could only be described as a time of "breathless expectation."

The memories came flooding back! "Breathless expectation" could easily describe the interminable wait until my next baseball game during my playing days, especially in Little League! It was pure torture! I would put on my uniform and have my glove ready to play hours before game time! Christmas! My older brother and I absolutely could not sleep on Christmas Eve; our excitement and anticipation were so great! Then there was the almost yearly "new kid in school" routine that I experienced as an "Army Brat." The expectation the night before was probably best described as anxious excitement, yet the unknown was still present. It was not fun being the new kid.

Over time, these experiences gained more significance. The day before I entered West Point at the age of 17 remains etched in my mind as if it were yesterday! I thought I had an idea of what to expect on that first day, but I soon realized I had no clue. It was immeasurably more difficult than I ever imagined. After four years filled with hard work, perseverance, and literally my blood, sweat, and tears, graduation day arrived, and the anticipation of that day truly left me breathless. This was soon followed by my first assignment with the Army in Germany, my acceptance into medical school, the birth of our first child, graduation, the start of my residency, and finally, its completion. However, the most intense memory remains the night before I deployed with the 101st Air Assault Division to Saudi Arabia for the First Gulf War. It was, and still is, the worst day of my life, leaving my wife and our three young sons without knowing what would happen next or if I would return. That night, my wife and I lay in bed, holding each other and crying. It was a painful moment.

What were the times in your life that you would describe as "breathless expectation"? A more pointed question, though, would be, "When was the last time you felt this in medicine?" I would bet that early in your careers, this experience was not uncommon - the first day of medical school, the first patient interview, the first blood draw, the first IV, the first case presentation, the start of residency, or the beginning of clinical practice. Do any physicians, or for that matter, any health care provider, experience this anymore once the "newness" of medicine wears off and the daily grind of medicine begins?

Wouldn't it be great to experience that feeling again? To have so much excitement about what tomorrow will bring that we are breathless with expectation - we can't wait for the next day to come! Many would say that's no longer possible in today's chaotic, unpredictable, and volume-driven healthcare culture. The optimistic side of me disagrees. I believe you can have those moments, but only if you take the time to step back, reflect, and remember why you chose medicine, why what you do is important, and that you make a difference in people's lives every day. The sacred relationship between physician and patient is the catalyst for those times of "breathless expectation" that once kept us awake at night with excitement and anticipation.

CHAPTER 21

"Wow!"

"Wow!" the child's voice echoed from the theater's farthest corners—a single word that everyone heard. The orchestra had just completed a stunning performance, and before the audience could burst into applause, that small, innocent voice articulated what everyone felt—their souls had been touched. The Conductor heard it, too, and it brought him to tears. He anticipated enthusiastic applause, perhaps a standing ovation, or even an encore request, but a genuine exclamation like this from a child? Never! That one word, spoken spontaneously and with reverence, is what all musicians strive for: to move someone so profoundly that their very soul exclaims, "Wow!"

He resolved to discover that voice, that singular individual. He yearned to convey his gratitude for bringing him joy, a joy he had forgotten. After weeks of searching, he found it. It belonged to an eight-year-old boy. However, this was no ordinary boy; he was profoundly autistic and, remarkably, non-verbal. His parents had never heard him speak until that very moment! The Conductor was left speechless, tears filling his eyes once more as the extraordinary nature of that moment became vividly apparent. It affirmed for him that his work held significance and purpose in a way he had never completely grasped.

I reflected on my own "Wow!" moments—witnessing the births of my children, the vibrant hues of a sunset or sunrise over the ocean, awe-inspiring snow-capped mountains, sunlight dancing on a clear, flowing mountain stream surrounded by a brilliant tapestry of autumn colors, and the stunning beauty of a rainbow trout. When did you last experience a "Wow!" moment? That moment when you exclaimed in wonder at something so beautiful and moving that you couldn't help yourself. It's in these extraordinary times that your humanity, the caring, compassionate essence of who you are, becomes more vivid and personal. When these moments arise, the inner child, often forgotten amidst years of education, work, and life's demands, awakens once more. Make sure to acknowledge these moments for what they truly are: a precious gift and a heartfelt reminder that there is so much more to life beyond medicine.

CHAPTER 22

Sunrises and Sunsets

Turning 60 felt weird, unlike any birthday I'd experienced before. I thought to myself, "SIXTY! Am I truly 60?" Where has the time gone? Reflecting on my past, I see how much of it I had "wished away." We can all fall into this trap. Life presents challenges to face and tasks to complete in order to achieve our ultimate dreams. However, we often discover that our best years were spent fixated on the goals ahead. By doing this, we overlook the importance of appreciating the journey along the way.

I'm a passionate fly angler. I'll fly fish anytime, anywhere, and under almost any condition! In my early days, I fished from dawn until dusk, navigating over boulders, bypassing waterfalls, and wading through rough rapids in pursuit of the next trout. Over the years, while my enthusiasm for fly fishing remains, my perspective has shifted. It's no longer about the number of trout I catch or their size. Now, it's all about the experience—standing in a cold, clear mountain stream with my fly rod, casting to rising trout while enjoying nature's beauty, watching sunlight dance on the water, and witnessing a bald eagle swoop down to catch a trout. I take the time to pause, soaking in the surroundings and truly enjoying the moment. I even sit at the stream's edge and, I admit, enjoy a cigar! For me, fly fishing transcends simply catching fish, just as life is more than a destination or goal we relentlessly pursue.

I have accomplished many things in my life and still have many more I wish to pursue. One of my priorities, as odd as it might sound, is to witness as many sunrises and sunsets as I can. I can't recall the last time I missed either. This tradition began during a challenging phase of my life. Coffee in hand, I cherished the early morning's stillness as the sun rose and painted the sky with magnificent colors, nourishing my soul. It gives me a chance to reflect, meditate, pray, and appreciate everything around the plants, flowers, trees, and birds. In these simple moments, I find joy and tranquility. Ralph Waldo Emerson once said, "The Earth laughs in flowers." Life is too precious and fleeting to ignore the Earth's laughter in flowers and the beauty of sunrises and sunsets. May each of you discover your own "sunrise and sunset"; may you find the peace, contentment, and joy that nurture your soul.

What you do matters. Your actions make a difference. What you do is still a privilege. Thank you for being who you are.

CHAPTER 23

Grieving

"Grief never ends... but it changes. It's a passage, not a place to stay. Grief is not a sign of weakness, nor a lack of faith. It is the price of love." - "Anonymous"

The "price of love" is what we are now facing with Debbie's passing this weekend. As I write this, I am filled with grief. The entire hospital and all who knew Debbie are grieving. We have the right to grieve, and we must grieve. This is the cost of having loved her.

Even amidst heartache, pain, and loss, we could not have chosen differently. To not grieve would mean denying the impact of knowing Debbie. That would be the greatest loss of all. Not having known her heart, witnessed her smile, or experienced her love for others would mean missing out on "The Dance". I would choose to partake in the "Dance of Life" with Debbie, with all the grief that follows, over never having known her and missing everything she offered, of which there was so much!

Being in medicine means experiencing grief, pain, and heartbreak intimately. These feelings become all too real for us. Over time, we develop hearts like "stained glass windows" — shattered yet beautifully reassembled, stronger for having been broken.

Debbie's life had a profound impact, touching countless individuals in unique and meaningful ways. May we aspire to live a life of such meaning.

The cherished "Mr. Rogers," who influenced many childhoods, once said:

"I believe that appreciation is a holy thing - that when we look for what's best in a person we happen to be with at the moment, we're doing what God does all the time. So, in loving and appreciating our neighbor, we're participating in something sacred."

Thank you, Debbie, for having a heart like a "stained glass window." Thank you for showing us how to appreciate the best in others. Thank you for teaching us how to love others. Loving you came at a significant cost. Our grief may never fully subside, but it will transform, and we will be changed for having traversed this journey.

Well done, Debbie; may you rest in peace. We love you.

CHAPTER 24

What Makes You Cry?

Growing up, I seldom cried. The most memorable occasion was when I was twelve, pitching in the semifinals of the Tennessee State Dixie Youth Baseball tournament for a chance to qualify for the Dixie Youth World Series. In the first inning, I allowed a walk and two hits, including a three-run homer. However, I pitched the next five innings without giving up any hits or runs, ultimately striking out 15 batters. Despite my efforts, we lost 3-2, and I cried. My tears were for the loss and the end of my dream to go to the World Series. However, more importantly, I cried because right after the game, I got in the car with my family to leave for my father's next Army assignment in Ft. Leavenworth, Kansas. We went straight from the field to Kansas, and I never saw my closest friends or the best baseball coach I ever had (even through college) again. Such was my childhood.

When I was nine and again at fifteen, my father served in Vietnam, experiencing significant combat both times. Despite knowing the risks, I didn't cry when he left. I was raised with the notion that "Men don't cry," which translated to me as "Boys don't cry" either, so I suppressed my emotions as best I could. Movies like "Old Yeller," "Shenandoah," and the book "Where the Red Fern Grows" didn't help, either! I was skilled at concealing my tears.

For thirty years, I didn't understand that it was acceptable for men—myself included—to cry. This realization came from another man, Lloyd, with whom I spent many years on mission teams. I got to know him even better than my own brothers, and I love him like a brother. Lloyd exemplifies the idea of a "man's man." He excelled in sports during college and was even drafted by the Montreal Expos. Yet, he was different from any man I had ever known—he cried openly and without shame. He wept for the needs and suffering of those we encountered on our missions and when he witnessed God's work in others. Before long, I found myself crying too.

While listening to classical music, I found myself contemplating writing this story. The sweeping crescendos and decrescendos of the movements, along with the delicate touch of piano keys or expertly played string instruments, resonate with my soul and bring me to tears. I find myself moved by the beauty of a sunrise or sunset over the ocean, by mountains towering above a clear, shimmering stream, and by my son playing with my grandson. I also reminisce about the precious moments shared with my sons long ago. These experiences impact me profoundly.

What brings you to tears, if anything does? You've likely experienced moments filled with joy or faced heartbreak and tragedy. It's not about gender; it reflects the state of your heart and your own humanity. I know your hearts. They have become like "stained-glass windows," once shattered but now mended, stronger and more beautiful than before due to their brokenness. You know this truth well. It's the "cost" of healing, a price worth paying. So, what makes you cry?

CHAPTER 25

The Missing Link

Medicine is challenging and becoming increasingly so, a reality you understand very well. Numerous factors contribute to this. Yet, one essential element, when absent, drains the joy from practicing medicine. That missing link is passion—specifically, a passion for your daily work. Without passion, joy evaporates, and what remains is merely labor: hard work that feels less fulfilling, meaningful, and enriching to the soul. The growing demands and expectations continue to press down, slowly extinguishing whatever joy is left.

Where does this passion originate? I believe it stems from a dedication to something greater than oneself. This commitment influences your identity and actions, aligning them with a purpose beyond personal interests and direct benefits. It transforms your perspective from being self-focused to being others-focused, shifting from a selfish heart to a selfless one.

In the absence of this passion, enduring the inevitable low points in life becomes incredibly challenging, if not impossible. During these times, you might experience feelings of being a "dead man walking," merely going through the motions as you struggle to get through another day, all while feeling unnoticed by others. You dig deep within yourself for the resilience to carry on. This strategy may offer temporary relief, but eventually, you risk depleting your inner resources, leaving your "bucket empty."

I understand what it means to live devoid of hope and joy. I've faced my own "valley of tears," teetering on the brink of despair and hopelessness. Each day becomes a struggle for survival. Where is the joy, the satisfaction, the meaning in this? However, embracing a cause greater than oneself can ignite a passion that fuels strength and purpose to keep going.

Without such a commitment, the uncomfortable question emerges: "Is this all there is?" Regardless of your appearance or how much wealth, fame, power, or status you possess, you will confront a profound sense of unfulfillment, incompleteness, emptiness, and even suffering. Joy evaporates, and the passion for your pursuits fades into a distant memory.

To overcome this crisis, it's essential to have a commitment to the future, to a purpose that instills a passion for living and the accompanying joy. Every individual possesses the ability to make this choice. By doing so, you will rediscover passion, energy, and joy. You will experience a life that matters, one that creates impacts in ways you can hardly imagine. I have made this commitment, and it has transformed everything! What might such a commitment look like for you? Moreover, how would it influence you, your family, your friends, and those around you?

CHAPTER 26

You Are Not an Island

The years 2000 to 2002 were particularly challenging for me. I served as President in a bustling Internal Medicine private practice, where my outpatient clinic was so full that I couldn't accept new patients. Hospital call was managed the traditional way, prior to the era of Hospitalists, meaning I worked 24-hour shifts for both assigned and unassigned patients, followed by seeing patients in my outpatient clinic. I typically spent my nights on hospital call in the hospital. Returning home proved pointless, as I would inevitably be called back for an admission. Additionally, I faced numerous phone calls from the answering service or floor nurses. The demands of the call were intense and growing. Alongside this, I was actively involved in the church, engaged in medical missions, and coached my sons in baseball and basketball, all while striving to be the best husband and father I could be. I was not doing a very good job as a father.

Any of these factors could elevate stress levels. However, the breaking point came with my mother's diagnosis of a rapidly progressive form of myelofibrosis in early 2001. At just 66 years old and previously healthy, this news was devastating. The year 2002 proved to be the hardest. My father, three brothers, and sister struggled to cope with her illness and the impending reality of her death. Unfortunately, my mother's hematologist and oncologists did a terrible job communicating with them.

As a result, I unintentionally became "her doctor" in my family's eyes when all I truly wanted was to be her son.

From January 2002 until her passing in May, I would leave my office as early as possible on Fridays to drive 7 ½ hours to my parents' home in Alabama. I did this to visit my mother, reassure my family, and ensure she received proper care. Each Sunday, I returned home, only to repeat the same routine week after week, month after month. The only exception was when I was on call. Needless to say, this was emotionally and physically exhausting.

I began to notice a change in myself that I initially struggled to comprehend. I became increasingly irritable, impatient, and withdrawn, to the extent that upon entering an exam room to see a patient, I felt an almost overpowering urge to leave. It became a challenge to remain in the room and listen to the patient's complaints, especially as my own life circumstances made their grievances seem trivial. I started to question whether choosing a career in medicine was a mistake. I was definitely experiencing "burnout," among other things, though I had not fully acknowledged this yet.

One night while driving to Alabama, I was searching for a radio station as I passed outside of Atlanta. I stumbled upon a talk station discussing depression, particularly in men. Surprisingly, I found myself compelled to listen; as I heard the description of how depression manifests differently in men compared to women, I realized that I was experiencing nearly all of what they described! I was not just "burned out" or had made a wrong career decision. I was truly clinically depressed! The thought of depression had never crossed my mind. After all, I could handle stress as well as anyone. My years at West Point, my time in the Army, including a war zone, the arduous years of medical school and residency training, more than proved I could handle anything, or so I thought.

Upon returning from Alabama, I promptly sought help. More importantly, I began confiding in close friends for the first time. Until that moment, I had kept everything to myself, attempting to cope on my own. I believed I could manage it alone as I had successfully done in the past. I quickly improved; my irritability, impatience, and frustration faded away, and I returned to my usual self.

From this experience, I realized that no one is exempt from major life stressors and the potential repercussions, such as burnout, disruptive behavior, maladaptive reactions, and even depression. I had underestimated the likelihood of this impacting me; I thought such issues were confined to others or my clinic patients. Yet, it did happen to me, and it can also happen to any of you.

There is a saying, "No man is an island," and it holds great truth. People require support, encouragement, and assistance from others during challenging times. Recognizing this need is not a weakness; it reflects wisdom. Failing to acknowledge it can lead to severe emotional and physical consequences for both yourself and your loved ones. Help is accessible, whether it involves talking to a trusted friend or seeking professional assistance. I understand the demanding nature of your work, which is becoming more challenging. Please take care of yourselves so you can do the same for those entrusting themselves to you.

CHAPTER 27

"This Is Water"

"There are two young fish swimming along, and they happen to meet an older fish swimming the other way, who nods at them and says, "Morning, boys. How's the water?"

And the two young fish swim on a bit, and then eventually one of them looks over at the other and goes, "What the hell is water?"

These are the opening lines of the renowned author David Foster Wallace's final book, "This Is Water," published shortly after his passing in 2008. He poses a question to university graduates: "How do you measure the value of the education they received?" What follows is a thought-provoking exploration of what he terms "the capital-T Truth." Wallace argues that the challenge we all encounter in grasping this "capital-T Truth" lies in overcoming what he refers to as "your default setting." This is the mindset you revert to when faced with life's challenges. It represents the automatic, often subconscious belief that something is true, even if it's incorrect. Why is this the case? Because, to some degree, we all think of ourselves as "the absolute center of the universe, the realest, most vivid, and important person in existence." Anything outside of that perception is often disregarded or unrecognized, much like the young fish who didn't comprehend what water was, as their inherent default setting failed to distinguish it from themselves. Their worldview was entirely self-centered.

Wallace argues that our tendency to view situations solely from our perspective, while dismissing other potential viewpoints, has led to remarkable wealth, comfort, and personal freedom in contemporary society. He describes it as "The freedom to be lords of our tiny skull-sized kingdom, alone at the center of all activities." However, he contends that the "most precious" kind of freedom is rarely discussed, particularly in a culture that emphasizes winning, achieving, and showing off. This more valuable freedom entails attention, awareness, discipline, effort, and a genuine ability to care for others, often requiring repeated sacrifices. Haven't we all made similar sacrifices for others throughout the challenging years of education and training, and even beyond?

Do you find yourself living in "your default setting," unaware of what is genuinely real and significant (like the young fish's question, "What is water?")? Or do you consciously choose a life that recognizes what is essential yet often overlooked, reminding yourself repeatedly, "This is water. This is water."? By doing this, you gain that "precious freedom"—the ability to truly care for those entrusted to you. You can then do what you do best, better - making a difference in others' lives with daily compassion and care.

Life is precious, the work you do is important; and your impact on others can be transformative. Let not the demands and frustrations inherent in medicine distract you from what truly matters, the reason you chose this path, and the difference you make each day. What is my "capital-T Truth"? It's about leading a life that matters, making an impact on others whenever I can. What's yours?

CHAPTER 28

What Are You Passionate About?

"What are you passionate about?" This is a question I often ask people when I meet them for the first time. Anytime I am around young people, as I am through medical missions, I always ask this question. I believe the answer to it is key to understanding the heart of that person.

We can be passionate about one thing or many things. I bet if asked, every one of you could quickly come up with an answer to this question. If you cannot, you should ask why not, because one's passions, to a significant extent, reflect who they are as a person, emotionally and spiritually. Who wants to live a life devoid of passion? I cannot imagine doing so. To me, that would be a life without adventure, without purpose, without real significance—a boring life.

I have my passions. The passions that define who I am as a person. Those who know me understand that I am a passionate fly-fishing enthusiast! I will fly fish anytime, anywhere, and under almost any condition. Additionally, I tie my own flies and craft fly rods. My enthusiasm for this hobby is immense! Standing in a cold, crystal-clear stream with the mountains all around me brings me complete peace. My thoughts are solely focused on catching the next trout and expressing my gratitude to God for letting me experience such beauty. I can easily fly fish for hours without thinking about anything else—none of the work obligations, life pressures, or current troubles—just the tranquility, beauty, and joy of the moment and the trout!

As passionate as I am about fly-fishing, it does not compare to what truly excites me - leading short-term medical missions around the world and investing in, mentoring, and encouraging young people. I have had the privilege of leading over 40 medical missions to eight different countries on four different continents since 2005. I have served alongside hundreds of amazing people who share a passion for serving and loving others. They want to live a life that counts, a life that makes a difference in the world. They are also our future, and they want someone to mentor them, to invest in them, and help them through the ups and downs of life. That is what I do, that is what I am passionate about. My question again is, "What are you passionate about?" How do your passions affect your life priorities, who you are as a person, and even as a physician, or do they?

Every hospital must have a "Culture of Excellence", a culture that is passionate about exceptional patient care. Anything less should not be acceptable. This is a passion worth having! The humbling thing is that each of you, whether in the hospital or outside, is doing this! What you do every day for your patients, your hospital, and your community makes a difference and is foundational for providing this exceptional care.

As always, thank you for all you do every day on the front line of patient care. I know the hard work you do, and I will never forget it. You are making a difference - one life at a time.

CHAPTER 29

Speedy

In 1972, I was 17 and a senior on the football team in Alabama. It was the third game of the season, and we had a standout halfback named "Speedy," who was black. Our high school was relatively well integrated at the time, thanks to its proximity to a military base. However, most of the schools we faced were still largely segregated. Racial identity defined individuals, and that night, the ugly reality of racism manifested on the football field. The week before, our school had received hate letters brimming with racial slurs, threats of injury, and even death. They specifically warned us not to bring our "n****s," in short, Speedy.

Early in the third quarter, we were ahead, and Speedy was having a great game. Despite the previous threats, it had been a hard-fought but fair game up until that point. Then it happened. As a defensive player, I was on the sidelines when Speedy sprinted past for a 20-yard gain. Just five yards from where I stood, he was shoved out of bounds. As he lay on his back with the play halted, another player from the opposing team lunged at him, colliding headfirst into Speedy's helmet. He did not get up. The coaches rushed to his side, and after several minutes, he was taken away in an ambulance. We ended up losing the game.

We didn't hear anything more until the next morning when the coaches called our homes. Speedy was dead! Disbelief and shock immediately followed, soon giving way to anger. The threats had escalated beyond mere words. As a team, we reviewed the game film and "the hit", rewinding and replaying that tragic moment. We all felt that it was intentional, that Speedy had been targeted. We sought action, justice, and revenge. However, nothing was done; there wasn't even a penalty for the late hit. In Alabama's world, it was merely seen as an unfortunate accident, just part of the game. I cried, we all cried, and our lives were changed forever.

Why share this story if it doesn't directly relate to medicine? I share it to provide insight into who I am, both as a person and a leader. Someone who detests prejudice and injustice. I write it so that those too young to remember that era of history may understand how far we've come, yet recognize how far we still have to travel. I write because life is invaluable and tomorrow isn't guaranteed. I write because Speedy's story still needs to be heard.

For anyone interested, this story appeared in the October 14, 2013, issue of Sports Illustrated. It can be found at SI.COM/speedy by scrolling down to the link titled "The Ghost of Speedy Cannon," where you can also view the hit on a segment of the 16mm game film.

CHAPTER 30

A Cry from My Heart - A Letter to a Journalist

Dear Sir,

"I'm not entirely sure why I feel the need to write to you. You might not even read this email, but I still feel compelled to do so. I am a 56-year-old Christian white male physician residing in North Carolina. I graduated from the United States Military Academy at West Point and the University of Alabama School of Medicine. Growing up, I was an "Army Brat" since my father was a career Infantry officer with two combat tours in Vietnam. I am also a veteran of the First Gulf War.

My upbringing was in a conservative, deeply Southern environment. My mother's family hails from the mountains of North Georgia, while my father's roots are in rural Mississippi. My ancestors fought for the Confederacy. Though raised in a loving and supportive family, I was surrounded by the prejudices of the era, resulting in my earliest experiences being shaped by an environment of racism. I am a product of the Jim Crow era.

For many years, I have followed your column in the local newspaper. To be honest, I often found myself either cursing you for your words or crying as I recognized their truth. There were numerous times I hesitated to read your articles because I anticipated they would only upset me, yet I still did. Why? Because your words cut through my heart like a scalpel, skillfully removing the lingering hatred, racism, and prejudice deeply embedded within me. Thus, I continue to read your work, and just yesterday, I found myself compelled to write to you. I'm not quite sure how to put it, but I NEEDED to reach out to you.

I appreciate your honesty, even though it can be brutal and challenging at times. There are moments when I feel like discarding your articles after reading them; however, I refrain because they provoke thought, evoke emotions, and occasionally bring me to tears as I come to grips with the ongoing hate, evil, and injustice of racism in this nation—a nation I love and once vowed to defend, a commitment I would gladly uphold today. I wish I could claim that the racism of the past no longer exists, but I cannot. Are conditions better than those dreadful times of the Jim Crow era? I believe they are, but do they align with where they should, ought to, and must be? The answer is clear, and Dr. Martin Luther King's dream remains distant.

Two significant experiences transformed me as an individual. After many years in the Deep South, where most Infantry bases are located, my father received a new assignment at the Presidio of San Francisco in the summer of 1969. I was not yet 14, and for the first time, I was confronted with the harsh reality of my own prejudices.

Then, Joey Robinson entered my life. He was among the most popular kids in high school, a standout athlete, and he was black. Despite my being a tall, skinny, shy, awkward kid with glasses, large ears, and a pronounced Southern accent, Joey accepted me for who I was. We became close friends, and through him and other black classmates, I began to realize how misguided my earlier beliefs about "colored people" truly were in my still relatively short life.

I will never forget the last time I saw Joey. It was the summer of 1972. I was moving the next day to Alabama, as my father had been given a new assignment. Joey and I attended a San Francisco Giants vs. Atlanta Braves baseball game. After the game, we returned to my home and said goodbye. I never saw Joey again, though to this day I miss him. What I remember most about that day, though, was not the game but my mother saying goodbye to Joey. Joey had become part of our family. My mother hugged and kissed Joey as she tearfully said goodbye. After Joey left, my father looked at my mother and said, "I never thought I would see the day that you would kiss a black man." To her, to all of us, Joey was neither black nor white; he was "us" - he was me, I was him. (Where are you, Joey Robinson?)

Months later, I am in my Senior year in high school - quite a culture shock going from California to Alabama! I am a member of the high school football team. The school is well-integrated, and relations between blacks and whites are good, considering it is Alabama in 1972. The presence of a nearby Army post helped, as black students from military families are very much the norm. Our team captain is an amazing young guy with the appropriate name of Speedy. He was our star halfback, the Junior class President, and he was African-American. Everyone loved Speedy!

Not only was he an amazing person, but he was also an excellent student, a true leader, and a friend to everyone.

Early in the season, we were scheduled to play a team from a part of northern Alabama known for its racism and continued presence of the KKK at that time. The week of the game, my high school and the football team began receiving hate mail from the town where we were to play. The mail, as you would expect, spewed death threats and racial epithets - we were not to bring our "n****s" with us.

Speedy, in particular, was targeted. We went anyway.

Early in the third quarter, we were ahead, and Speedy was playing brilliantly when tragedy struck. Speedy executed a sweep to the right, gaining 20 hard-earned yards. He was knocked out of bounds just 5 yards away from me (I played defense, so I was on the sideline). As he rolled onto his back well past the boundary, the referee called the play dead. An opposing player sprinted in, launched himself, and collided with Speedy head-on, helmet to helmet. It was a clearly late, deliberate hit. Speedy lay there, motionless. He was rushed to the nearest hospital, and that night, we received the devastating news that he had died from a severe brain injury and a bleed. The following day at practice, we all gathered as the coaches repeatedly showed the film of the hit that took Speedy's life. We mourned deeply for him, and this tragedy forever changed us all.

I share this because I am tired of the racism, covert and overt, that remains embedded in our culture and, yes, in our hearts. It will not disappear quickly. It will take the passing of those raised in such a way and the raising and education of the "next generation". I now realize that my anger is not directed at you. You make me think, you make me question, you make me look deep into my heart, and when I do, I see the racism that still exists. I am angry, but not at you, rather at myself, and it hurts, and I cry. I will continue to read you and, as I do, I pray God will continue to transform me into a person who simply desires to love God and others."

Author's Note: I wrote this in 2012 to Mr. Leonard Pitts, the Pulitzer Prize-winning journalist with the Miami Herald, in response to one of his commentaries in the local paper.

CHAPTER 31

A Matter of Honor

A few years back, I attended my 40th West Point class reunion. It was a fantastic experience, particularly reconnecting with friends I lived, studied, and trained alongside during those challenging four years. We genuinely were "a band of brothers". Even 44 years later, my time at West Point plays a crucial role in shaping my identity today.

During the reunion, I was interviewed by West Point's Center for Oral History due to my experiences as a cadet, specifically during the Honor Scandal of 1976. This significant event garnered national attention and threatened the very foundation of West Point's Honor Code. Although I was innocent, I found myself entangled in the situation, fighting to prove my innocence and defend my honor. Instead of being presumed innocent until proven guilty, I faced the presumption of guilt until I could demonstrate my innocence. It was a harrowing and transformative period.

The honor scandal revolved around an electrical engineering exam taken by my entire class shortly before Spring Break during my junior year. Although it was a take-home test, we were honor-bound, as with all work at West Point, not to ask for or receive any assistance from anyone— no matter how minor. Failure to comply requires that you footnote any assistance received, resulting in a corresponding reduction in your grade. For reasons known only to them, many of my classmates opted to assist one another without acknowledging that help. Consequently, they violated the code. An extensive investigation followed.

In the following months, I was moved, along with others who were under investigation, to a designated barracks separate from the rest of the Corps of Cadets. I was relieved of leadership responsibilities within the Corps for the summer, assigned a lawyer, and given a trial date. When I first met my lawyer, he informed me that I had just a 20% chance of being declared innocent. I was utterly taken aback. I replied, "Sir, you're suggesting that someone who is completely innocent has only a 20% chance of being found innocent?" He pointed out that, until that moment, many of my classmates had gone before the Honor Committee and all had been found guilty and dismissed. It was the lowest, darkest time of my life. Being falsely accused is one of the worst things that can happen to a person.

My lawyer became convinced of my innocence, leading to a lengthy battle to prove it. I ultimately won, but it took a significant emotional toll. I felt deep resentment toward West Point and everything it symbolized—an institution boasting over 200 years of exceptional education, military training, leadership development, and character building. However, I, along with many innocent classmates, became entangled in an investigation that resembled a witch hunt. In the end, hundreds of us were scrutinized, resulting in over 150 being found guilty and dismissed, leaving a rift within my class that remains largely unhealed to this day.

Graduating was a bittersweet experience for me. I was overjoyed to have endured the hardships of my four years, yet I couldn't shake my bitterness toward West Point. As I drove through Thayer Gate into "freedom," I purposely tilted my rearview mirror up, avoiding any glimpse of it. I was so upset that I refused to wear my class ring for years, questioning whether my experience had been worthwhile. Over time, the painful memories began to fade, and my anger subsided. Upon my acceptance to medical school, I recognized the vital part West Point had played in that achievement, leading me to realize that all the suffering and sacrifices had indeed been worth it.

Having endured that challenging period, I have become a better person. Consequently, I've developed a strong sense of justice and a commitment to embody honor and integrity, following the West Point motto "Duty, Honor, Country." As a leader, I strive to foster a culture of respect that empowers individuals to do what they do best, better, and realize their full potential!

CHAPTER 32

Getting Personal

I once spoke at a Leadership Forum focused on Opioid Abuse, specifically addressing the role of hospital systems in tackling this vital issue. Reflecting on my talk, I realized I had very little new to contribute; the crisis has reached epidemic levels, and hospitals are poorly equipped to take proactive measures. It feels insurmountable.

Through my experience leading medical missions, I acquired a crucial insight that shifted my perspective. The world's needs can also feel overwhelming, but they only become tangible when they touch us personally—you must live it, breathe it, taste it, smell it, and touch it. In 2009, the opioid crisis became personal for me; it transformed into a reality I could not ignore.

As a physician leader, I prioritize transparency. It is essential for fostering a safe and compassionate culture where others feel empowered to emulate such openness. In an environment marked by transparency, remarkable outcomes can occur! I hope my "Bugle Notes" over the years have conveyed this commitment to transparency effectively.

When I decided to write this book, after considerable thought and prayer, I also made the choice to be open with my readers. This choice makes me feel exposed and vulnerable, but I choose to proceed regardless. My hope is that by sharing my story, this crisis will resonate more personally with you, making it feel more real. This narrative recounts how close I came to descending into the dangerous realm of opioid addiction (or any addiction, for that matter). I was fortunate enough to halt my journey before venturing too far down that road. Sadly, many are unable to stop and find themselves trapped in a downward spiral toward the deep, dark abyss of despair and its companion, hopelessness. If this can happen to me, it can happen to anyone. If my story helps even one person avoid this fate, then the anxiety I feel in sharing it will be worthwhile.

It started following my first back surgery in 2009 for a severely herniated disc during a medical mission to Moldova in Eastern Europe. The pain was excruciating, the worst I had ever felt. My right leg was weak and numb, forcing me to be carried into my host home and laid in bed—there was no running water, a rudimentary outhouse, and sporadic electricity. The conditions were far from ideal. I resorted to taking prednisone, hoping it would help. But the following morning, I was no better, in fact, worse. As the team leader, I realized I would have to be urgently evacuated to the U.S. However, a "miracle" occurred that allowed me to regain neurologic function temporarily, and I was able to finish the mission. That "miracle" may need to be the topic of another "Bugle Notes"!

Two days after I got home, I underwent surgery, which turned out to be completely successful. I was sent home with a prescription for OxyContin, along with a refill, a routine practice at that time. It effectively managed my post-operative pain and surprisingly made me feel quite good overall, providing a calming effect as well. Before my mission trip, I had been dealing with significant stress from home, my practice, and the hospital. I started to look forward to taking it. Since I was still on medical leave, I didn't worry about it impacting my patient care; I could simply enjoy the feeling at home. I convinced myself that this was perfectly fine and that I could quit whenever I wanted. I had no idea I was heading down a dangerous path.

Each day, I found myself counting the remaining tablets, dreading the moment they would run out. It embarrassed me to think of calling the neurosurgeon for another refill, fearing he might view me as an addict or drug seeker— something I believed could never happen to me. But soon, reality hit. After using the last pill, I developed withdrawal symptoms within 24 hours: restlessness, abdominal cramps, and diarrhea. Though these symptoms were relatively mild, they frightened me. I never thought I'd become physically and mentally dependent; I believed that only "weak" people or those lacking "self-discipline" faced such issues. I was mistaken.

The experience was both surreal and frightening, as well as humbling. It felt surreal because I never imagined it could happen to me, and humbling because it revealed my vulnerabilities. This experience provided me with a fresh perspective on people who face addiction in any form. If it can happen to me, it can happen to anyone! Nobody is immune.

Many of our colleagues are at risk, if they aren't already in a downward spiral. The stresses in medicine can lead anyone to seek an escape, and substance abuse is a common avenue. I genuinely care for each of you and hope you avoid falling into this alluring trap, as the repercussions can be devastating. Therefore, I share my story with uncertainty about how you will react—whether it will alter your perception of me or raise doubts about my capability as a leader. My sincere hope is that my experience makes this crisis feel more personal and tangible to you. Only then can you truly understand the challenge ahead and devise the best ways to confront it.

CHAPTER 33

A Legacy - What Will Be Yours?

As I near the end of my medical career, I feel the need to pause and reflect. Memories rush back—thousands of night calls, tens of thousands of patients cared for, those who passed away, the joys, the heartbreak, the doubts, the burnout, the tears, and the hugs; the good times and the bad, the joyful moments and the sad ones. I can't help but wonder how I will be remembered and what my legacy will be.

There are several things I hope to be remembered for:

- I lived a life that mattered, making a difference for God, my country, my family, my community, and the underserved of the world.

- I experienced the world's needs personally, making them real to me.

- I was a physician who cared for the whole person, doing so with excellence, humility, and a servant's heart.

- I invested in, taught, encouraged, and mentored the next generation—our future—whenever I could

- I was a servant-leader, caring for people and inspiring others to do what they do best, better.

- I worked to bring joy back into medicine because, without joy, medicine is just hard work.

- I lived a life that reflected West Point's motto: Duty, Honor, Country.

We will all leave a legacy. The past is history from which we learn and grow. The present is here and now. This is the time to lay the foundation for your future years. When you come to the twilight of your life, how do you want to be remembered? There will be no second chances or go-backs.

SECTION II
SACRIFICE

CHAPTER 34

Sacrifice

"Those things which are precious are saved only by sacrifice."

-Private First Class David Kenyon Webster, one of the first recipients of the Purple Heart.

The Purple Heart was established in 1782 by George Washington to honor soldiers who were killed or wounded in action, or who suffered as prisoners of war. It represents the sacrifices made by countless men and women throughout our history. The preceding quote deeply resonated with me as I reflected on my own experiences during the First Gulf War, particularly the immense difficulty of leaving my family without knowing what lay ahead or when I would be home again. The hardest day of my life was when I departed Ft. Campbell, KY, for Saudi Arabia. I wept openly as I bid farewell to my wife and three young sons, ages 8, 5, and 2.

Sacrifice can appear differently to different individuals. Olympic athletes selflessly commit years to train for competition at the highest level. The sacrifices of the "Greatest Generation" should inspire humility in all of us. They endured the Great Depression and then fought in a brutal war that took many away from home for extended periods, while their families patiently managed the home front and awaited their return, often with great anxiety. Nearly 500,000 did not make it back.

My father completed two combat tours in Vietnam while my mother worked hard to raise my siblings and me. Each night, we set up TV trays and watched the evening news, eagerly looking for any glimpse of my father as the latest film footage of the ongoing combat played before us. The ringing of the phone struck deep fear in my mother, an experience I'll never forget, even though I was just 10 at the time. Too often, a phone call brought heartbreaking news—the ultimate sacrifice paid, once again. My mother made the greatest sacrifice of all.

Each of you is well acquainted with sacrifice. Years of intense study, coupled with extensive training, have made this experience all too familiar. You have dedicated time, resources, and your personal lives—including marriage and family—to reach this point. Thank you for the sacrifices you have made in the past and for the ongoing contributions you provide daily in service to others. I express my gratitude, as does our community, and most importantly, our patients appreciate your efforts. Always keep in mind that your work is significant; what you do makes a difference every day, and it is a privilege to do what you do. You are our "most precious" resource, and your sacrifices have been worth it!

CHAPTER 35

Soldiers and Fathers

In his 30s, he was strikingly handsome with short-cropped hair like a soldier's. This was Ukraine, engaged in war with Russia. He was now part of that war, one that the rest of the world seems to have forgotten or lost interest in, even as its young men continue to face the harrowing realities of the front lines. His unit's chaplain reached out to me because he had just returned from the front after many months. Each year, he brings "his boys", who are still healing from both physical and emotional scars, to see me. Given my own experiences in war, I could at least listen to them with empathy, and be a source of support and encouragement.

The animosity towards Russia is palpable. Given Ukraine's history under the USSR's hegemony, this reaction is understandable. However, this animosity is deeper and more pervasive, piercing to the soul. Every soldier's death intensifies it, fuels it. Males aged 18 are required to serve for three years and often find themselves on the front lines, as was the case with this soldier. He had served with bravery and distinction even though he wasn't a front-line combatant; he was the Music Director for his unit! Yet, the front lines were fluid and unpredictable, with no truly safe area. He often found himself nearly encircled by Russian soldiers. He started to carry a "big gun," stating, "If you are captured by the Russians, you never return." I sat shocked.

He recounted his experiences with calmness, detailing a severe concussion from an artillery explosion, numerous shrapnel wounds, and the deaths of three fellow soldiers killed beside him while trying to reach safety. I noticed no signs of obvious emotional distress. I chose to inquire about his adjustment back home with his family. Tears filled his eyes as he revealed that the only reason he was alive was his family. His wife and two young daughters were constantly in his thoughts and prayers. He was resolved to survive for them at any cost.

As I listened to his stories and gazed into his eyes, I started to envision my father as I will always remember him—big, strong, and the Airborne Ranger Infantry officer he was. He, too, had faced combat and lost many men, including some close friends. Yet, he returned home from that war twice, seemingly unscathed by it all. Memories began to emerge from a deep place within me. That's when I recalled that my father had died exactly one year ago today. I had spent those last two weeks with him, the memory still painful.

The tears came. I thought of my sons, now grown. Had I truly been present for them? How many moments of their lives had I missed while caught up in the demands of medical school, residency, service in the Army and the First Gulf War, and establishing my practice—all the busyness that is life? The lyrics from Harry Chapin's song "Cats in the Cradle" echoed in my mind:

"And the Cat's in the Cradle and the Silver Spoon,

Little Boy Blue and the Man in the Moon."

"When are you coming home, Dad?"

"I don't know when, but we'll get together then, son, you know we'll have a good time then."

These words served as a guiding compass throughout my life. Despite missing much of my early years to war and other assignments, when my father was home, he was fully present. My happiest memories are of throwing the baseball with him. I vowed never to allow those haunting words to manifest in my own life. I would do as my father did. I would be present.

I looked at him, this "ghost of my father" seated before me, and said, "Go home, hold your wife, tell her you love her. Return to your girls and tell them they are beautiful, they are smart, and they are important". He nodded, tears running down his face. He reached for his right shoulder, took off his unit's combat patch, earned through immense cost and sacrifice, handed it to me, and walked away. My interpreter and I were left stunned. She, too, was in tears.

I needed solitude—to reflect and to mourn. I found solace wandering the dirt paths of the beautiful village of Ostap'je, with a light snowfall gently covering the freshly plowed fields, ready to nurture new life.

Guard yourselves against wishing time away amid the distractions of your busy lives, in the search for something more or better. Time is precious, time is now. It will slip away too quickly, taking with it memories that reside deep within us. What you do is hard. I understand. I care. Thank you for caring as well.

CHAPTER 36

They Saw It in Color

I recently rounded in the hospital on a 100-year-old veteran of the Battle of the Bulge. It was a terrible and costly battle fought in Belgium during the winter of 1944-1945, the coldest and snowiest in memory at that time. The German army made a desperate last stand against an increasingly powerful US force, resulting in hundreds of thousands of casualties. He experienced it firsthand; it's not just a forgotten memory frozen in time in a black-and-white photo. He saw it in color. His account prompted me to reflect on the other stories I've heard from different patients.

He began to cry. I quickly apologized, assuring him he didn't need to respond. After regaining his composure, he stated it was alright. He was a veteran of D-Day, June 6, 1944, serving as an infantry private with the 9th Infantry Division. He was part of the sixth wave that landed on Omaha Beach on that fateful and blood-soaked day—a day that altered the course of history. I can hardly imagine the horrors he witnessed as he stepped off the landing craft into what could only be termed hell. I inquired about his most vivid memories from that day when he was just 19, fresh out of high school. He replied:

"I remember my best friend from high school was just a few yards away when we landed. Within seconds, he took a direct hit by an artillery shell and was blown to pieces."

He began to cry again. I asked no further questions.

He served as a door gunner on a B-17 with the 8th Air Force, which carried out bombing raids over Germany. During the war, two-thirds of the planes, each with a crew of ten, were shot down. Tens of thousands of American lives were sacrificed. To return home, you needed to survive 25 missions, a challenge most couldn't meet. His plane was shot down on what was supposed to be his next-to-last mission. Most of the crew managed to parachute to safety, only to be swiftly captured and taken to a farmhouse, where they were lined up against a wall.

He was standing next to the pilot, the "old man" of the crew at age 23. A German officer walked up to the pilot, drew his Luger, and without saying a word, shot the pilot in the head. He then turned and walked away. My patient spent the remaining months of the war doing hard labor in southern Germany, working in a mine.

He was one of the original Navy "Frogmen," the predecessors of today's Navy Seals. He was part of a team whose job was to swim to the Normandy coast under the cover of night, hours before the D-Day invasion was set to begin. Their mission was to secure closely guarded bridges critical to German resupply and troop transport. It had to be done silently. They used their knives to accomplish this mission.

I write to remind you, as the patient mentioned above reminded me, that this "Greatest Generation" will soon be gone. It will be a sorrowful day when the last of them passes away. I had the honor of caring for many of them. I wanted to hear their stories. I NEEDED to hear their stories before they could no longer be told. I can't help but wonder how many stories I missed and are now lost forever?

The joy of medicine, for me, stemmed from cultivating trust-filled relationships with my patients. They would share their stories, allowing me to see glimpses of their lives when they were youthful, strong, and capable. Eventually, only black-and-white photos from the past will be left. For them, though, they saw it in color.

So, take the time now, while you can, to hear your patient's stories.

CHAPTER 37

Words of Appreciation to Nurses

This "Bugle Notes" is dedicated to every nurse. Over the nearly 40 years since I began medical school, I have had the honor of working alongside countless nurses in both hospital and outpatient settings, as well as during over 40 medical missions I've led globally. Additionally, there are five extraordinary nurses in my family. Each nurse I have collaborated with has taught me valuable lessons, helping me become a more compassionate, caring, and empathetic individual, as well as a better physician. I unabashedly tell people how much I love nurses for who they are as people and for what they do as nurses.

I have reflected on what the "things" are that make nurses truly special. Not everyone possesses the qualities required to be a nurse. Certain attributes characterize those who opt for nursing. In my experience, these qualities often align with those of physicians, yet there remains something inherently unique about individuals who pursue nursing that differentiates them. I want to share my reflections, which come sincerely from my heart. I hope every nurse who reads this will feel inspired, empowered, and appreciated for who they are as a person and for what they do as a nurse.

You are the frontline of healthcare, spending the most time each day with our patients and their families, addressing their personal, physical, emotional, and spiritual needs.

You are the eyes and ears of the patient; you serve as their greatest advocate. You must have the clinical acumen to identify potentially serious problems with a patient and the confidence to make it known to the physician. I know that is not always an easy thing to do.

You have a servant-heart - humble, loving, and caring. The needs of others always come first to you.

You are able to notice the need around you and go to that need, whether it is a patient or a co-worker.

You wear many hats - mediator, negotiator, peacekeeper, and at times, the voice of truth when patients and their families are frightened, angry, vulnerable, feel forgotten, or alone.

You are "hope-givers" when there seems to be no hope. Without hope, life loses its meaning.

You are the "warmth of love" given through a caring touch, a gentle hug, or a comforting word precisely when it is most needed.

You are a difference-maker in the lives of people every day, and you do it one life at a time.

You are "right there with them" during a patient's and their family's greatest time of need.

Finally, when all else fails, and there is nothing medically left to do, you are the "tears of a loving God" when a patient has no one else to turn to in their grief and sorrow.

Mother Teresa once said, "None of us do truly great things, but we can all do small things with great love."

Every day you do just that – you do the small things with great love, and in doing so, you are making a difference in the lives of all you touch.

Being a nurse means possessing a heart "like a stained-glass window"—a window that has been broken only to be forged back together, stronger and more beautiful for having been broken. Thank you for having such a heart! You are a blessing to those you serve and to every provider fortunate enough to work alongside you.

"You are beautiful, you are important, and you are loved."

CHAPTER 38

The Wait

February 24, 1991, and I wait. I sit on the edge of my cot beneath the pitched canopy of my distant canvas home; its sides pulsating in the ever - present wind; sand seeping through the walls, everything air-brushed a pastel tan, outside the vast Saudi Arabian desert, limitless in every direction. The winds of war have been blowing and the time has come. Ten of us are in the tent, all physicians waiting, all far from our homes and families, all pondering the same questions – What will it be like? Do I have what it takes? Will I remain steadfast and perform my duties as Blackhawk helicopters blacken the sky with wounded soldiers? The First Gulf War has commenced. Operation Desert Shield has now become Desert Storm.

I am the Chief of Medicine for a 400-bed Army field hospital located just south of the Iraqi border. For months, we have meticulously planned and prepared to receive over 600 casualties each day, transported directly from the battlefield by the Blackhawks. Nurses, Corpsmen, and Technicians have been cross-trained to do whatever is required so the doctors can be where they are needed the most. I bear the responsibility of triage—a weight that feels tangible, and the questions come.... I write to my mother and father and tell them I love them. I reflect on how my father, a combat veteran of two tours in Vietnam, did what he did, and I wait.

Decades later, I wait again. We are once again at war, this time against an unrelenting, invisible, and merciless foe—a virus that has never been encountered before; there is no immunity; it is a pandemic. COVID-19 has become part of our everyday vernacular. We hear daunting projections— millions infected, hundreds of thousands dead; it's surreal, incomprehensible, unprecedented. What is true, what is not? What to do; what not to do? I think of the doctors, nurses, physician assistants, nurse practitioners, and hospital staff who are now on the front lines, in harm's way, waiting as well, grappling with the same questions I faced so long ago.

Many are my friends. The "peak" has yet to arrive, and we continue to wait. For me, the waiting is the hardest part. Yet soon, this waiting will end, and when it does, the questions will be answered, and "new heroes" will emerge. Let's thank them now as they wait and fight.

CHAPTER 39

Sacred Trust

The words "sacred trust" evoke a response within me that I find difficult to put into words. However, it is clear, as all of you understand, that a "sacred trust" undeniably exists between a doctor and a patient. This trust is the glue that holds a healing relationship together. It is a privilege granted to us by patients and their families when they allow us to engage deeply in their lives through this remarkable bond.

Patients, in their most vulnerable state, open up to us, disclose things to us, in ways very few professions experience. They may reveal details they've never disclosed to anyone else. They consent to invasive physical treatments because they trust, hope, and believe in us. Sacred trust is essential for establishing a genuine healing relationship. Without trust, there can be no relationship; without a relationship, there is no special bond that transcends all the forces driving healthcare transformation. In the absence of this sacred trust, the true art of medicine is lost, along with the joy it brings.

Many transformational forces are currently impacting healthcare. What will become of this sacred trust? Will the future model for medicine be based solely on algorithms that provide a treatment plan drawing on the latest clinical evidence, gleaned from a massive database? This model requires no human interaction, relying solely on analytics.

Increasingly, it appears that this is the direction medicine is heading. However, such a model misses the critical human element of healing, caring, and compassion. It lacks intuition and judgment. It also completely ignores the art that is medicine.

Medicine is both an art and a science. This sacred trust must exist in a healing relationship as well as in science. The transformative forces influencing healthcare should enhance, not detract from, this relationship. People want a human connection in their care. To achieve this, a framework for healthcare delivery must be established to show how these transformative forces can strengthen the healing relationship. This is the challenge for healthcare leaders today. This is why we, as physicians, must reengage in all aspects of healthcare and lead the way through this transformation.

How will this look? I don't know. I am not sure anyone knows at this point. Changes are happening at an astonishing pace, and we must be prepared to tackle this challenge. Central to all of this is maintaining that sacred trust. The relationships we forge with our patients—and the sacred trust that emerges—are the primary motivations for many of us in medicine. Without it, our roles become mere jobs: hard work devoid of joy. You make a difference every day, and this sacred trust is one reason why.

As always, thank you for the many sacrifices you have made and continue to make to ensure our patients receive the best possible care in a loving and compassionate way.

CHAPTER 40

A Servant Heart

As I prepared for my next medical mission, I began to think about the word "minister." Obviously, from a religious standpoint, it has certain connotations, one of which is "to serve". When you are ministering to someone's needs, you are serving them.

This brought to mind my dear friend in Nepal, Fahad. He was a young Muslim physician with whom I had the privilege of collaborating during my first two medical missions in that region. I will always remember our first day serving together, working side by side. Over four and a half days in the clinic, we saw just over 4000 patients, many of whom had significant physical and medical needs. It was overwhelming, especially with only eight providers available to assist them!

The first day proved to be particularly challenging as we hadn't expected such a large influx of patients. The weather was extremely hot and humid as well. By day's end, we were all both emotionally and physically drained. It was then that Fahad approached me with tears in his eyes, sharing words I'll always remember: "Dr. Andy, I have never seen people like you. My entire life, I have been told to take care of myself, work hard, and prepare myself so that I could be successful. Then, if I have time, I could help others. But today, watching you and the team, I am learning that I am to put others' needs before my needs, to serve others first!" I was utterly astonished by this. He grasped a lesson in one day that many individuals never come to realize or understand.

Servants have a servant-heart—one that is loving, obedient, and humble. People understand the concepts of being loving and obedient, but grasping humility, the act of showing humility, can be more challenging. Often, humility is mistaken for timidity, passiveness, or even weakness. The reality is that humility is not any of those! In my office, I have framed on my wall a definition of humility that I compiled from various sources. I display it prominently as a constant reminder of how I should be. It says:

"Humility is not timidity. It is not an attitude toward ourselves. Rather, it is an appreciation of other people. It is a respect for them as persons of worth, a recognition of their abilities, a willingness to receive from them what they have to offer.

We clothe ourselves with humility by helping others do what they are capable of doing and by recognizing their successes. We do so by listening rather than talking to them. We do so by supporting them rather than competing with them. We clothe ourselves with humility, in other words, by putting others ahead of ourselves."

Every day in the hospital and in your practices, when taking care of patients, healing them, comforting them, you are ministering to them. You are serving them. You are putting them first. You are a servant with a servant heart, and I am most grateful for you!

CHAPTER 41

Ten Commandments of a Servant Leader

I have observed both excellent and poor leadership. As a leader, I have also made my share of mistakes, and I am certain I will make more. When that happens, I will promptly take responsibility, learn from the experience, and do everything possible to avoid repeating the same error. Nonetheless, there may be occasions when I fail to recognize my shortcomings, which can occur with any leader. This brings attention to a crucial point: leaders must be held accountable.

My leadership style is rooted in servant leadership, which was instilled in me during my time at West Point. Many years ago, I developed what I refer to as my "Ten Commandments of a Servant Leader." These commandments are grounded in my life experiences, lessons learned, wisdom gained, and my personal faith journey. Each week, I review a checklist of these commandments to assess my adherence, thus ensuring I remain accountable. My "Ten Commandments of a Servant Leader" are:

1. People are your most precious resource; take care of them

2. "Clothe yourself with humility"

3. Eat and sleep last (Your people's needs come before your needs)

4. "Open wide your heart" (Being transparent)

5. Trust is the foundation of all relationships

6. Make a difference each day, one life at a time

7. Encourage, teach, and mentor every chance you can

8. Every day is a good day, and some days are better than others! (Having a positive attitude)

9. Listen more and talk less

10. Learn to follow

"If serving is below you, then leadership is beyond you."

-Anonymous

CHAPTER 42

A Band of Brothers and Sisters

"We few, we happy few, we band of brothers; For he today that sheds his blood with me Shall be my brother; be he ne'ar so vile,

This day shall gentle his condition; And gentlemen in England now a-bed

Shall think themselves accurs'd they were not here And hold their manhoods cheap while any speaks That fought with us upon

Saint Crispen's Day."

William Shakespeare's "HENRY V"

In Shakespeare's "HENRY V," prior to the Battle of Agincourt (1415), King Henry's battered army, significantly diminished by both combat and dysentery, finds itself cornered by a formidable French Army that has cut off the sole escape route to England. The French knights, clad in heavy armor and exceptionally skilled, seemed destined for victory over the English forces. In this moment of despair, King Henry V delivered a powerful address to his remaining troops, famously known as the St. Crispen's Day speech. The final lines of this speech have become widely recognized as "The Band of Brothers" speech. Through his words, King Henry V inspired the English Army to achieve victory!

You are a "band of brothers and sisters" just like those men were centuries ago. United, you face a formidable enemy—one that seems daunting and where victory may not be guaranteed. This enemy is the ongoing transformation of health care, with all its associated changes and uncertainties. Other unknown challenges will surely arise in the future.

The safety and well-being of our patients have never been as important or as challenging as they are today. Patients are older, sicker, and more complex, yet advancements in technology have enabled us to do much more for them. The sacrifices you must make have also never been greater—long hours, night calls, emergency surgeries, critically ill patients, dying patients, and demanding families, along with the never-ending administrative and EMR responsibilities. It would be easy to feel overwhelmed and give up, just as it might have been for the soldiers at Agincourt. Yet, you continue to make a significant impact on the lives of others; you are living a life that truly matters! Isn't that how we all wish to be remembered—having lived such a life—while so many others will think themselves "accurs'd", that they cannot say the same?

CHAPTER 43

A Decision Made

Three straws held in a hand; each varying in length; a decision to be made. It was September, 1990, the hospital commander arranged them to appear equal. The instructions were straightforward: the longest straw wins. However, the consequences were severe—separation from family, enduring physical and emotional challenges, potential injury, and even death. We were three Army physicians assigned to the hospital at Ft. Campbell, Kentucky, staring at the straws, the weight of the decision heavy in the air. One of us would remain behind, the choice falling to whoever drew the long straw. I ended up drawing it, meaning I would stay while my two colleagues deployed with the 101st Air Assault Division to Saudi Arabia for Operation Desert Shield, which would soon transition into Desert Storm, marking the First Gulf War.

I sat still, grasping the long straw. Initially, I felt relief. I wouldn't have to leave my wife and three young boys to face potential danger. I glanced at my partners. One was just two months out of his residency training and was newly married, his eyes cast down, shoulders hunched. The other was experienced, like me, and also had a young family. Suddenly, memories of my father flooded back. It was summer 1965 in Ft. Benning, Georgia. He was preparing his gear to deploy to Vietnam with the 1st Cavalry Division, marking the first major escalation of the war. He appeared joyful, while my mother was anything but. His humming and whistling only made her angrier. I recall her saying, "Why are you so happy? Don't you know you could be killed and leave me with all these children?" I can still hear my father's response: "Don't you understand that this is what I have trained and prepared for my entire life?" In that moment, I realized I had to go. I couldn't stay behind. I had also prepared and trained for war since my time at West Point. A decision was made; my new colleague remained behind.

Decades later, another crucial decision looms. The coronavirus has emerged, a pandemic has been declared, and the uncertainty remains unsettling. For me, this feels like a war; it's different from my first experience, yet still a war. This time, the adversary is unseen. The media is rife with hype. What's true and what's not? What should we do or avoid? This novel virus brings with it countless questions and a toll on human life—a perfect storm for fear. I remember the straws and my father's words. I can't remain passive while others, physicians, nurses, and hospital staff, face danger. They are my friends, colleagues, my "band of brothers and sisters." Together, we've navigated challenges, dedicated to caring for others regardless of the situation. I've made my decision: after five years in hospital administration, I will return to patient care. I have to; my father's voice echoes in my mind.

CHAPTER 44

Fahad, My Friend

I received a phone call last night, and it was not just any call but from Nepal, a place dear to my heart. Nepal is where I love the beautiful and humble people, the exotic culture, the simplicity of life, and the towering mountains. Not just any mountains, but THE MOUNTAINS—the Himalayas with Everest looming above them all. Now, Nepal is fighting for its very existence after a devastating earthquake. Does 'catastrophic' even come close to describing the current situation? I lack the words to fully depict the rubble in Kathmandu or the hundreds of once-beautiful mountain villages now buried under "mountains" of boulders and dirt—homes shattered and buried; homes where they were born, raised families, and planned to die—but not on that tragic day. How many more "thousands" of men, women, children, and entire families are still unaccounted for, and is the worst-case scenario becoming reality?

I have led many medical missions to Nepal, walking through Kathmandu's narrow, bustling streets filled with pedestrians, cyclists, and motorcycles. Only the smallest cars can navigate these passageways. Everywhere, an intricate maze of electrical wires crisscrosses from building to building, creating a chaotic web. Many structures seem on the verge of collapse. Despite the chaos, I walk shoulder to shoulder with the crowd, feeling confined and pondering, "what if... ?" Then, the "what if" becomes reality. I can see, smell, taste, touch, and hear everything that makes Kathmandu unique. It's an incredibly exotic city — in my eyes, the most fascinating city in the world. And yet, now...

The phone call! It was from Fahad, someone I've known since my first mission to Nepal in 2009. I've grown to love him deeply over the years. He was one of three young Nepali physicians who volunteered to work with us, all just finishing their first post-medical school training year. Two were Hindu and one was Muslim, Fahad. Despite knowing we are a Christian organization, they still wanted to support us in any way they could. I welcomed them with open arms, as did the entire team, and in the ensuing week, we grew to love them deeply, but especially Fahad.

We worked tirelessly over nearly five days, attending to more than 4000 patients. Our small team consisted of only 12 Americans, five of whom were medical providers, along with three Nepali physicians. Every morning, we arrived at our temporary clinic- a tiny, one-room church - and faced a line of 500 to 600 people. Most had traveled hours or even days by foot, donkey, or oxcart filled with hay, to see the "American Doctors," whom they believed could fix anything. Few had seen a doctor before. When ill, patients typically either recover on their own, survive with lasting, often debilitating complications, or die. The nearest hospital was hours away, accessible only to those with money. Sadly, this has been my experience in nearly every country I have served. We were overwhelmed by the physical, emotional, and spiritual needs. Our hearts broke, tears shed, prayers lifted, and hope shared. That day, the world's needs became truly personal to me.

Fahad, my friend, was right beside me, caring deeply for his people. Coming from a more privileged background, he had never ventured into this part of his country—the poorest region in one of the world's poorest nations. Although he had encountered poverty before, it was never as intense as this. Who among us can say otherwise? Yet, he endured the relentless oppressive heat, with the sights, sounds, smells, and sickness all around us, making it deeply personal for him too.

I will never forget that moment. We finally saw the last of nearly 800 patients that first day, and we were exhausted—beyond exhausted. It was the kind of exhaustion that follows the worst of the worst call days, only more intense. Fahad came up to me, crying. He said words that I will always remember, words that bonded us forever as brothers despite our completely different worlds.

"Dr. Andy, I have never encountered someone like you. Throughout my life, I was taught to work hard, study diligently, prepare for the future, and prioritize my needs. I believed that doing these things was essential to becoming a respected doctor and achieving a good life. Today, watching you work, I realized how mistaken I was. I have seen how much love this team shows to every patient. I have observed the compassion and care emanating from your hearts, and most importantly, I have seen how you put the needs of others before your needs. I understand now that I, too, must follow your steps. I must prioritize the needs of others over my own. I am to serve others first, their needs always before mine."

I was speechless! In a day, he learned a life lesson that most people never learn: we are to put the needs of others before our own. I told him that God had transformed his heart and given him great wisdom. I told him that he was right. It is in the serving of others, in the placing of others before ourselves, that we become a complete physician, not just the facade of one.

Fahad is safe, but my heart aches as I hear him describe the death and suffering he endures daily. The grief, sadness, fear, and even anger are evident. While his family remains safe, it was days before he heard from his best friend, Ambesh, who also served with Fahad and me during that initial mission.

Ambesh was alive but had lost his sister, her husband, and their young daughter. Fahad was devastated, crying as he shared this with me. He hadn't spoken to Ambesh yet because he couldn't bring himself to call him. He was afraid. What would he say? He worried he might become speechless, not knowing the words to say. What would I say in such a moment? I wanted to comfort him, but the thousands of miles between us prevented it. I assured him I loved him, would pray for him, and was there for him, but those words felt trivial compared to the harsh reality he faced.

Fahad, in moments like these, who truly knows what to say? Often, there is no need for words. Simply being there for him—holding him, crying with him—can be enough. As Christians, we believe that Jesus, during such times, "is the tears of God for us." You can become that for those you love who are hurting. No one can fully understand what Ambesh is experiencing unless they've gone through similar pain, heartbreak, and despair like he and many others in Nepal are enduring now. That's why words often fall short. Sometimes, just showing him love and being present is enough. Call him, Fahad. He needs to hear your voice and know that he's not alone, even if he feels alone right now. Tell him that your heart is breaking for him, that you love him (and yes, it's okay for a man to say that!), and that you are there for him.

He said he would call him and thanked me for my advice.

Yesterday, he sent me a picture. Beneath the picture, he had written," Wanted to share this. It's beyond me to describe. I can only wipe my tears." The picture was that of a young Nepali mother, dead, lying on her back. Her son, probably 6 months old, was alive, lying naked on top of her, suckling at her breast.

Tears escaped my eyes. How could they not? I replied to him, "My eyes and heart cry for you, my brother. I am so sorry you had to witness this. As hard as this is to see, this needs to be seen. The world needs to know the pain and suffering that is now Nepal. BUT... I reassure you that Nepal will rise up from the ashes and your generation will lead it. Please keep sharing your heart with me.

As my wife and I climbed into bed, we thanked God for our many blessings, as we always do. Then it hit me, do I really appreciate, do I really recognize how blessed I am, or do I simply go through the motions of living life with all its busyness and, as an afterthought, each night, simply repeat without comprehending the words, "Thank you, God, for all our blessings"? I am certain tonight will be different. May this day and every day be different as well for each of you. May your blessings be truly heartfelt. Please keep Nepal in your prayers and thoughts. If you knew the people like I know Fahad, your heart would be broken, too.

CHAPTER 45

Nurses

This week is "Nurse Appreciation Week," and I want to share this "Bugle Notes" to express my sincere appreciation for all nurses. Oddly enough, the first thought that came to mind when I learned about Nurses Week was my first day at my very first military assignment, just months after graduating from the United States Military Academy at West Point in June 1977. I was a new Second Lieutenant, often called a "Butter Bar" in military slang. How this connects to nurses will become clear soon, so please bear with me!

I remember that first day as if it were yesterday. It was December 6, 1977. I had arrived in Zweibrücken, Germany, three days earlier. I was incredibly naive and nervous! My job was to be the Operations Officer for a Signal Communications Company supporting all US Army units in that part of Germany. I had no idea what the job involved or how to perform it. To increase my anxiety, I had three Non-commissioned Officers (NCOs) working under me. I was now their "superior" officer. Each NCO had between 15 and over 20 years of Army experience and knew their jobs well. Even more stressful was the fact that all three were Vietnam veterans.

Graduating from West Point is quite similar to finishing medical school. In both cases, you gain a lot of new knowledge and skills, but when it comes to applying that knowledge in the real world, we soon realize we know nothing, at least that's how

I felt in both circumstances. I bet most of you reading this felt the same on your first day as an Intern. Now, here I am, on my first day as the "new Lieutenant," responsible for all telecommunications, microwave, satellite, and telephone operations for a company of over 100 people supporting thousands of soldiers across southwestern Germany, and I know absolutely. nothing, zero, zilch.

However, and this is a big however, I at least understood that I knew nothing compared to other new Lieutenants going through the same process, who genuinely believed they knew everything and were determined to prove it to you. In medicine, the equivalent is starting as an Intern, where you can either admit you know nothing about patient care or pretend to know everything.

Only a fool would choose the latter, but just like in the Army, medicine is also susceptible to such foolish beliefs.

Being wise enough to know that I knew nothing and that these three NCOs now working for me were highly experienced, I chose the humble approach, saying, "I know nothing and I need your help." I entered the office where all three, in their late 30s to early 40s, were sitting, and at just 22, I said, "Hello, I am Lieutenant Andy Lamb, your new Operations Officer, and I know nothing about what to do or how to do it. I need you to teach me everything you know, and I promise to listen and learn. I cannot do this without your help." From that moment, they quickly took me under their wing and taught me everything I needed to know, plus more. Over the next 18 months, we grew very close, and I remain grateful for their willingness to teach and support me. I was their "superior" officer, but most NCOs see new Lieutenants as a nuisance unless they have the right attitude, as I did. When a Lieutenant approaches with humility, NCOs will do everything they can to support and mentor. That's the hallmark of a good NCO, and why they are the "backbone" of the Army. Without them, the mission cannot succeed.

Now, to get to the heart of this story! I grew to deeply appreciate the three senior NCOs who looked after and protected me. Similarly, during my Internal Medicine residency, I quickly developed a strong bond with the nurses, especially those I had the chance to work alongside and learn from during the early, uncertain months when I still knew very little about patient care. I want to emphasize again, only a fool would believe otherwise immediately after medical school. I treated the nurses on the wards, ICU, and ED the same way I did the NCOs. I needed them to tell me if I was making mistakes or if I could improve. I actively wanted and asked for their feedback. With love, patience, compassion, and professionalism, they cared for and watched over me. They were as integral to my learning experience as any resident or attending when it came to learning what true, compassionate, and personal patient care looked like. I will always be grateful to those nurses. I will always remember how they cared for me on call nights when I was sick with fever and could barely stand but still had to cover the ICU. I will never forget the head ICU nurse looking at me and saying,

"Dr. Lamb, you go lie down in the call room here in the ICU and sleep. We will call you if we need you, promise."

And that is exactly what they did. I slept in the call room, and they did not disturb me one time, even though the unit had many sick patients. They took care of every patient, and me as well. For this and many more reasons, I will unabashedly say, "I love nurses!" and I truly mean it. They were there for me and cared for me every time I needed them.

To all nurses who are on the "front lines" of medicine, lovingly, compassionately, and competently caring for patients - you are the "backbone" of medicine, and I thank you for who you are and all you do! You are greatly appreciated, needed, and loved.

CHAPTER 46

"...and They Loved Me"

During the battle for Okinawa in 1945, thousands of American soldiers and hundreds of thousands of Japanese soldiers and civilians lost their lives. The fighting was fierce and horrifying. Amidst this carnage, acts of courage and sacrifice shone brightly, especially that of PFC Desmond Doss. As a medic and a Conscientious Objector, he was determined to serve his country without carrying a weapon, driven by his faith that he could not take a life under any circumstances.

He was deeply respected by his unit as his courage was undeniable. On one nightmarish night, following hours of ferocious combat leaving over one hundred American soldiers wounded atop a 400-foot cliff, Doss's bravery went "above and beyond the call of duty," earning him the Medal of Honor.

Under constant enemy fire, and protected only by darkness and the gunfire from the wounded he aimed to save, he lowered one soldier after another to safety using a rope. Despite being wounded himself, he kept returning, telling himself, "Just get one more, just one more." That night, he saved 75 men single-handedly. Many years later, Doss explained in an interview, "I wasn't trying to be a hero. I was thinking about it like this—if it were a house fire and a mother had a child in the house, what makes her go in?" "Love," he said. "I loved my men, and they loved me... I just couldn't give them up, just like a mother can't give up her child,"

Doss's words powerfully highlight a special bond forged through shared hardships and sacrifices. Despite war's horrors, survivors often speak of missing the close connection with their fellow soldiers. I understand this bond well, and I believe each of you does too. For me, it was with my classmates at West Point, in residency training colleagues, physician tent mates during Operation Desert Storm, and those I served with on medical missions. This unique, intimate connection transforms the unbearable into bearable and the impossible into the possible.

I suspect you experienced this during your medical training as well. Those years of grueling work and sacrifice were possibly the toughest of your life, but the friendships formed may very well be some of the closest you have ever had. You were there for each other. You depended on each other. There was an unmistakable, unspoken bond between you. I believe the bond continues today.

Every day, you serve alongside colleagues and a myriad of others—nurses, APPs, and ancillary staff—who share a common passion for providing exceptional healthcare.

The passion therein is the fuel that stokes the fire from which this bond is forged and then strengthened by the demands and expectations you face.

Why write about this? Am I naive to think it important? There is no metric for it, and it is not on the "scorecard". I write because what you are doing together, whether in the inpatient or outpatient realm, is important. You are making a difference in the lives of others every day, and it is still a privilege to do so. My hope is that you will "see and feel" the bond that connects each of you. It is this bond, and the one you have with your patients, that will sustain you in the years ahead. When nurtured, this bond will not break. Cherish these times, these friendships, this bond, for they are reminders that you are part of something much bigger than you are. As a result, you can do even greater things!

CHAPTER 47

Christmas Eve

Christmas Eve 1990, Saudi Arabia, a few miles south of the Iraqi border - it is cold and dark as I lie on my cot with my sleeping bag wrapped around me. The steady hum of generators fills the background while I listen to Pachabel's Canon in D minor on my cassette player. Rain pelts the tent I share with nine other Army doctors. The tent sides sway rhythmically with the wind, mirroring my heartbeat, creating a symphony of emotions playing in my mind.

Two months earlier, I, along with over two hundred soldiers, departed Ft. Campbell, Kentucky, heading to the Saudi desert as Operation Desert Storm prepared to launch. As Chief of Medicine at the 86th Army Evacuation Hospital based at Ft. Campbell, I watched my normal life vanish after Saddam Hussein invaded Kuwait. Following weeks of preparations and repeated delays, we finally departed, unsure of what awaited us or how long we'd be there. We only knew war was imminent, and that a dangerous man, who had already shown willingness to use chemical weapons, was a threat.

We arrived in Dharan, Saudi Arabia, where we spent the next two months preparing for the upcoming conflict. We stocked supplies, equipment, and medication. Physicians cross-trained nurses and corpsmen to ensure we could provide the best care for the expected 600 casualties each day, mainly from the 101st Air Assault Division. Many nurses were married to those soldiers. Would their husbands be among the injured or dead? That concern weighed heavily on everyone.

On December 23, we relocated the 400-bed hospital eight hours north to the Iraqi border using 112 flatbed trucks. We managed to set up the hospital by Christmas Eve evening. It was a bleak period; our only link to our families was through mail, as there were no phone lines, Internet, cell phones, emails, or Skype—only letters. How special every letter was! I wrote home daily, as letters were my sole connection to my family, home, and the hope of reuniting one day.

That evening, word came down from the 101st Command Center that a substantial armor (tank) unit of the Iraqi Republican Guard was less than ten miles north and poised to attack. At that time, we lacked a defensive perimeter and armed security. During the cold, rainy night and into Christmas morning, the Engineer Battalion from the 101st worked tirelessly to erect anti-tank barriers and dig deep trenches between us and the Guard. I stopped feeling sorry for myself when I saw what those soldiers were doing. How could I ever repay them except by ensuring that, if they needed our medical assistance, we would be there for them? This gave me a new appreciation for sacrifice and the meaning of being part of something much larger than myself. My outlook on life, my family, and my priorities changed significantly.

I know how hard you work, the frustrations you face, and the sacrifices you make. It is easy to lose "perspective" on what is truly important in life. Maintaining a good perspective is crucial as you undertake your work. It won't necessarily solve the problems nor remove the frustrations you face.

Remembering past challenges or hardships, though, can help you view things through a different lens.

Like those soldiers on the front lines working through the cold and rain on that dreary Christmas Eve, I thank you for the sacrifices you make and all you do to care for our patients. Just remember that you are greatly appreciated!

CHAPTER 48

Veterans

I am a veteran, as are my father and all three brothers. I have been to war, separated from my family, the danger real, living in the desert in a tent, the sand blowing through the walls, sleeping on a cot with cardboard boxes as furniture.

I know the feeling of lying on that cot in darkness, missing your family so intensely that it physically hurts. Silently, tears flow as you endure this solitude. I recognize the sacrifices of all veterans and those currently serving.

I know the pain of leaving behind your wife and three young children to serve in a foreign country, where the risk of not returning is real. I know what it's like to cry uncontrollably during that final goodbye, unable to stop no matter how hard you try. You find a place alone to cry until there are no more tears left and then you pick yourself up and do your duty. I know the sacrifice.

I know what it's like when your father leaves twice for war in a distant jungle, where he would personally engage in combat. I know what it's like to watch your mother cry whenever a soldier in his unit is killed, feeling her fear that he might be next. I know what it is like to fear that someone might arrive at your door with a message of condolence from the President. I know the sacrifices the families make.

I know the commitment, sense of duty, honor, and country that veterans and current service members uphold. They would willingly sacrifice everything and risk their lives for freedom, regardless of the cost. I know that feeling. I know the heart of a veteran.

I know the pride that comes with serving your country, doing your best because you realize how fortunate we are to live in this country. I know how quickly this can be lost if it weren't for veterans. I know because I have been there.

Duty, honor, country—these three words define the core of every military person, whether veteran or active duty. They shape who they are, who they can be, and who they will become. It is the soldier who hates war most of all, because they are the ones called upon to make the ultimate sacrifice.

All veterans understand this. Please take a moment to thank a veteran and reflect on the sacrifices they have made for you.

CHAPTER 49

Making the Unbearable Bearable

I once heard someone say they wanted to "make the unbearable, bearable." These words deeply resonated with me, not only because of my experiences in medicine and on the mission field but also through the passing of my father. Watching the compassion and care of the hospice team allowed me to see how they made "the unbearable, bearable" for my father and my family. These words now feel real to me because they have become personal.

When caring for your patients, you are doing the same for them. They arrive distressed, scared, and vulnerable, often unsure of how much longer they can endure. They seek relief from pain that feels "unbearable" to them and their loved ones. By dedicating unhurried time, offering a gentle touch, speaking comforting words, providing a reassuring hug, or simply being there with them, you help make what is unbearable feel more manageable.

I write these "Bugle Notes" to remind you that every day, you make a difference in others' lives, that your work is meaningful, and that it's still a privilege to do what you do. This reminder is always valuable. If you've experienced emotional or physical pain, or felt hopeless and despairing, you know how true the word unbearable is. It becomes personal. You understand how to make the unbearable bearable. When

130

you achieve this, you impact a patient's and their family's lives. Let this be a reminder of why you chose medicine.

Thank you for living a life that counts, a life that makes a difference in this world.

CHAPTER 50

"Just Another Day in Paradise"

I have led 12 missions to El Salvador and have grown to love the country, its people, culture, and natural beauty. I often refer to it as "mi segunda casa," which means "my second home". However, the harsh reality is that it is frequently ranked among the most dangerous countries worldwide because of the severe gang violence.

Two dominant gangs control parts of San Salvador and many towns across El Salvador. They are a constant and brutal presence in the everyday life of the typical El Salvadoran. These gangs emerged from a terrible civil war in the 1980s that caused over 300,000 civilian deaths. Afterward, thousands of orphans were left behind. Their only chance of survival was to band together as a "new family," leading to the formation of the gangs. Now, El Salvador is witnessing the next generation of gang members, many born and raised within the gangs themselves. This new generation lacks conscience and is brutal beyond compare, willing to commit any heinous act to maintain control, power, and instill fear among the population. They regularly demand actions from the El Salvador government, and if their demands are not met, swift and often deadly retaliation against the people ensues.

During my visits to El Salvador, I have always felt safe. The government and my local partners do everything possible to protect us. We are always accompanied by at least three armed national police officers, specially trained in gang activity, around the clock. When we travel, police vehicles escort us, leapfrogging to ensure we don't stop at intersections or in traffic, reducing the risk of being targeted. Naturally, the safest routes are chosen, and no precaution is overlooked. The police officers become an integral part of the team and are deeply appreciated!

My last mission to El Salvador, though, was an exception. Gang violence had significantly increased due to the government's refusal to meet their latest demands. As a result, the gangs chose to attack public bus transportation, especially in those areas under their control. The day my team of 69 people arrived in San Salvador, six bus drivers were killed. Fortunately, no passengers were. The next day, another driver was killed just blocks away from the hotel where we were staying. Another bus driver was later killed. We were traveling on the buses normally used for public transportation. Our guards were on high alert, and as a team leader, I took extra measures to ensure the safety of the team and our young high school El Salvadoran interpreters. Many of our interpreters had to drive home with their parents everyday through a territory controlled by gangs. Despite all this, we remained safe, and the mission was one of the best!

During the week, I had the opportunity to engage in a long talk with my host partner, Rene, a man I have known for over 10 years and who is like a son to me. I received an education in the mindset and activities of these gangs that shocked me to my core. For brevity's sake, I will not go into all the details of the terror tactics and brutality used by the gangs on the people of El Salvador. It is heartbreaking and incomprehensible. As a result, the members on this mission came back changed. The needs of the rest of the world had become more than real to them; they had become personal.

Imagine how I felt on my first day back at work when I had a brief encounter with a physician from the medical staff. I arrived early that morning, and as I approached the hospital's main entrance, I saw a doctor I've known for years leaving the hospital. He probably had been called for an emergency, looked tired, and wasn't in the best mood. I greeted him and asked how he was. As he reached his car, he replied, "Just another day in paradise." I was tempted to ignore it, but after my recent experiences in El Salvador and my years of leading medical missions, I couldn't help but respond. I told him, "If you had been where I just came from, this would be paradise."

I probably should have stayed quiet. Looking back, I have no regrets. Is any hospital, or even our healthcare system today, truly "paradise"? Of course not. Still, we are very fortunate to work in a healthcare organization that offers a beautiful workplace, advanced technology, excellent support staff, and a safe environment. There's always room for improvement, and I recognize that. However, for me, this environment feels like "paradise" when I think back on all I have seen and experienced.

I know how hard you work and the challenges you face every day. I have been there, too. Sometimes I needed to be reminded how fortunate I was to do what I did when I became discouraged or frustrated for whatever reason. My intent with this story is not to lay a guilt trip on anyone but to provide a gentle reminder that, yes, things could be worse and, in fact, for the majority of the world, things are far worse, unimaginably worse. In light of this, we do experience to some degree, "paradise" every day, whether we recognize it or not.

CHAPTER 51

The Helicopter

Imagine you're 19 years old, critically wounded and dying in the jungle of the Central Highlands of Vietnam. It's November 14, 1965. Your unit is outnumbered 2 to 1, and with enemy fire so fierce from 100 yards away, your commanding officer has ordered the Med Evac helicopters to stop coming in. You're lying there, listening to the enemy machine guns, knowing you're not going to make it out.

Your family is around the world, 12,000 miles away, and you will never see them again.

As the world blurs in and out, you realize this is the moment. Amidst the machine gun fire, you faintly hear a helicopter. Looking up, you see a Huey approaching, but it doesn't appear real because it lacks Med Evac markings. Captain Ed Freeman is on his way to you. Though he's not a Med Evac pilot and typically wouldn't perform such a mission, he heard the radio call and decided to fly his Huey into the gunfire anyway.

Even after the Med Evacs were ordered not to come, he's still coming. He drops in and sits there amidst the machine gun fire as they load three of you at a time on board. Then he flies you up through the gunfire to the doctors, nurses, and safety. And he keeps coming back, thirteen more times, until all the wounded were out.

No one knew until the mission was over that he had been hit four times in the legs and the left arm. He took twenty-nine of you and your buddies out that day. Some wouldn't have made it without him and his Huey.

For gallantry above and beyond the call of duty, Captain Ed "Too Tall" Freeman was awarded the nation's highest honor, the Medal of Honor.

My father was an Airborne Ranger Infantry Officer. He knew Ed Freeman. He, too, like "Too Tall" Freeman, and all those involved in what was the first major battle of the Vietnam War, the battle of Ia Drang, were members of the 1st Cavalry Division. They deployed to Vietnam in the summer of 1965. This battle is immortalized in the book "We Were Soldiers Once and Young" and the movie years later. I remember the time well. I was 10 years old, living in Ft Benning, GA. During this time, a new concept of battle emerged, known as air assault, which involved bringing soldiers directly into combat by helicopter.

It was a hard time for my mother. She was alone with 4 children under the age of 13, the youngest less than 3 months. She cried often, especially when she received word that the husband of another friend had been killed in combat. In our neighborhood during 1965-66, there was not a man around. They were all in Vietnam. At the age of 10, all I knew was that my father was fighting a war in Vietnam. I never seriously thought he would be killed. Why should I? He was invincible in my eyes. Every night, as a family, we ate dinner on TV trays. We watched the iconic Walter Cronkite as he discussed the latest developments in Vietnam, the black-and-white, days-old film footage flashing before us. We watched, hoping beyond hope, for a glimpse of my father, our eyes glued to the screen. We thought we saw him once.

As I reflected on this story, I wondered if I could have done what "Too Tall" did? What motivated him, or anyone else, to perform such brave, selfless acts despite great personal risks? I began to see a link between his actions and what each of you, as physicians, does. This connection is a unique bond formed through shared hardships in pursuit of a common goal, whether it's years of intense medical school or demanding residency training. Few experiences forge such strong bonds as shared struggles for a cause. I've felt this during my time at West Point, throughout residency, and even during the first Gulf War when deployed near the Iraqi border supporting the 101st Air Assault Division. This bond also stems from being part of something larger than oneself. For "Too Tall" and my father, it was their identity with the 1st Cav Division, and the resulting sense of duty to their fellow soldiers and country. There is an unwritten code among soldiers - NO ONE left behind! From these bonds, relationships are made, strengthened, and invariably trust grows.

I believe the most important part of being a physician (or any health care provider) is not the clinical acumen possessed (as important as that is) rather the relationships developed and the surrounding influences and qualities produced by those relationships. A culture built on such relationships is one of trust, respect, and caring. This is a culture that allows the best in every person to be realized. In medicine, it translates to every patient getting the best care possible, every time.

I really appreciate you for being willing to be part of something bigger than yourself, through which you can do even greater things and make a bigger difference.

CHAPTER 52

"The First 100 Yards"

You are 19 years old, standing in the muck and mud of the trenches of World War I. You are cold, hungry, filthy, and exhausted beyond words, but above all, you are afraid. It is a visceral fear that defies description, one that only those who have faced the horror of combat can understand. You are an American soldier, and this is your reality. You know what awaits you when the order is given to "go over the top"—the withering fire from rifles, machine guns, and artillery; a rain of deadly, hot steel that indiscriminately strikes flesh and bone, mutilating and killing those around you, and, as you now painfully realize, quite possibly you. Any sense of youthful immortality has long been erased by the horrors you have already witnessed.

Survive the first 100 yards, you keep telling yourself. If you can just get through those 100 yards, your chances of surviving the day increase greatly. In fact, the victory that day seems almost guaranteed. A mere 100 yards...it might as well be 1000. Knowing many of your "band of brothers" around you will die, and that you might die within moments, you still press on. The order is given, and you charge over the top, fighting nearly paralyzing fear with a single thought: survive those 100 yards. How? Why? Because you cannot do otherwise. You refuse to let your buddy down, those you've shared extreme hardships and terrifying moments with- the bonds no one else can understand. You must be there for them; you will be there for them at any cost.

"The first 100 yards" is a powerful analogy for facing one's fears, struggles, and challenges; for persevering and doing what has to be done despite the fear.

Each of us has faced, are facing, or will face our own personal fears. Maybe they aren't as terrifying as those of a soldier in combat, but they're still scary in their own way. How will we handle such fear? None of us really knows until we are in that situation. All we can do is prepare the best we can and remember that we won't be alone. Others will face them with us. We are not isolated from the rest of the world. We all need each other. This simple truth I learned at West Point has helped me through the toughest times.

SECTION III
MAKING A
DIFFERENCE

CHAPTER 53

The Couple

It was dark as we entered a crumbling stone building—a one-room 15' x 15' structure. No electricity, no running water, no amenities, we assume "we all have." I was leading a medical team to Moldova, the poorest country in Europe—a country I had come to know and love well. The team had finished a busy day in the clinic. Before going to dinner, I wanted to make a home visit to an elderly couple my host partner asked me to see. They were not physically able to leave their home, so a few team members and I went to them.

As my eyes adjusted to the flashlight cutting through the darkness, a foul smell filled the small room - the odor of urine and feces. My interpreter spoke in Russian. From the darkness, a feeble voice of a woman emerged. That was when I noticed the two elderly individuals, a husband and wife, lying in small, separate beds against the wall.

They were in their mid-to-late 80s, which was unusual for this part of the world. They appeared frail and emaciated, their bony hands clutching the bed covers to their chins in the cold room. He was bedridden and unable to sit up on his own. He was lying in his own excrement. How long had he been like this—days, weeks, surely not longer? His wife was not much different except that, with help, she could get out of bed and sit. Against the right wall was a small stone oven for heating and cooking, but there was no firewood to be found. The ashes

143

were cold. She could no longer cook. They were entirely dependent on others for help, but there were no others. They had no family; the children were either dead or lived far away, trying to survive themselves. The neighbors had little to offer, as they were in the same impoverished state. This is life in Moldova: hard, extremely hard, and for many, a life lived without hope of getting better.

The woman, with help, set up and, tears welling in her eyes, grasped my hand, repeatedly expressing her gratitude for my visit. She mentioned that no one comes to see them anymore and that they are truly alone. She shared her heartbreak over being unable to care for her husband. She kissed my hand once more and thanked me again, her eyes filled with tears, now streaming down her face. We all cried.

I turned to her husband and introduced myself. The smell coming from him was overwhelming. When was the last time he had been out of bed, taken a bath, changed clothes, or had clean bedding? He could not remember. The interpreter asked me to look at his backside, so we carefully turned him onto his side. His bedding was completely soaked with urine and smeared with feces. I was stunned by what I saw: a very large, deep, and obviously infected sacral decubitus extending to the bone, with the characteristic smell of Pseudomonas, awakening memories of past patients.

We gently repositioned him onto the dirty bed. They offered us their limited food. She apologized for the house not being cleaned. She cried more. My heart wept. I promised we would return the following day. As we stepping outside into the fresh air washing over us, we were speechless. What to do or say when faced with such unexpected misery, suffering?

144

Words were not adequate to describe what we had just witnessed and experienced.

The next morning, sunlight streamed through the window, and the scene before us was more devastating than we remembered. The couple reached out to us, weeping with joy, never imagining that we would come back as promised. Then, the real work began!

Everything and everyone were moved out of the house into the sunshine. Some team members cared for the couple, removing their ragged, soiled clothes and beginning the long process of bathing them. A tender act of love followed as the husband and wife, with gentle care, were washed until their emaciated bodies were finally clean. However, the decubitus was another issue. It was cleaned and dressed as best as possible. It was all we could do. In his world, there were no other options.

The house was scrubbed on hands and knees, removing human waste and caked mud that covered the floor and even along the walls next to the beds. One of my most vivid memories is my 16-year-old niece scrubbing the floor, wanting to do whatever she could to help. New clothing, mattresses, pillows, sheets, and blankets were purchased. Every necessary item we could think of was provided. After six hours of work, they were carried back into their "new home." They wept openly when they saw all we had done. We all held hands, prayed, and cried together.

I promised we would be back at the end of the day to check on them. We returned as darkness fell and were warmly greeted by them. Once again, though, the first thing we noticed was the smell of fresh urine. He had wet his new bedding and clothes. Of course, how could we expect otherwise? Yet, they were so grateful, so appreciative. They even tried to give us a gift from their meager possessions to thank us. We told them that they had already given us the best gift of all, the opportunity to love and serve them. In doing so we hoped that we had also brought them a small glimpse of love, kindness, and hope, something they had not had - in years?

A deep sadness washed over me. How horrible their lives must be! The truth is that much of the world lives like this—desperate, hopeless, and often alone. To live without hope isn't really living. Being alone without friends or family would be even worse. I know what it feels like to be hopeless, joyless, with no hope that things will ever improve. That leads to despair, which is painfully hard to describe unless you've been there. But loneliness? I have never truly experienced it. What must it be like to be both hopeless and alone? The truth is that many people live like this. Patients often come to their doctors in deep despair. I read a recent article about how loneliness in the US is increasing along with the emotional, spiritual, and physical toll it takes. Physicians, surprisingly (or maybe not), rank high in loneliness.

Loneliness, hopelessness, they are all around us, yet we are missing them! How many times have I missed it because I did not take the time to learn more about the patient I was seeing? How many times have you? There's much more to medicine than just the clinical side. Equally important is the human side. This is where the "Art of Medicine" takes place. This is where you are needed the most. Let's not miss it!

CHAPTER 54

Without Hope

"The only end to pain is the graveyard." Those words are etched forever in my mind. They underscore the hopelessness felt by so many throughout the world. She was 90 years old, crippled by arthritis, with no family, living alone in a dirt-floor hovel with no electricity or running water. She lived in a tiny village of 2,000 people in the poorest country in Europe— Moldova. She lived every day without any hope that her life would get better. Her entire life had been one of daily hardship and struggle to survive. She only knew the physical and emotional pain. She had no hope, no joy.

I was leading a short-term medical team to Moldova as part of a faith-based organization that sends teams to the poorest and neediest countries in the world. Moldova, in Eastern Europe, was once part of the Soviet Union. It is, though, for historical reasons, viewed by surrounding countries as the "ugly stepchild" of what is now Russia. Multiple factors through the years have contributed to this -oppression under communism, the "Great War" (known to us as World War II), the purges under Stalin and other Soviet leaders, corruption, and finally, the collapse of the Soviet Union, resulting in Moldova's complete economic and socio-political collapse. Moldova has not recovered, and life there remains hard.

Each day of the clinic, I would send a small team to make home visits. On one particular day, I went with the team.

Home visits in developing countries can be both powerfully moving and emotionally heartbreaking. As you go into the homes of the poorest of the poor, you never know what you will see, hear, or experience. More often than not, you leave that home changed by what you just experienced. Such was the case with this woman. She was thin and frail. Arthritis had crippled her body. She walked slowly, bent over, cane in hand. I sat with her on the concrete steps leading into what was her "home". Through my interpreter, we spoke of her health issues, trying to determine what could be done for her, if anything. Her only complaint was the arthritis pain that she lived with constantly.

As I sat with her, I noticed she was staring into the distance at a cemetery. Then she said those words: "The only end to pain is the graveyard." As someone who had lived nearly her entire life under communism, she had no belief in God or "anything more" after death. All she knew was the ever-present physical pain from arthritis and the emotional pain of loneliness. Her only hope of ending this pain was death—the graveyard.

I remember vividly thinking how terrible it must be to live a life without hope—any hope. That was the only life she knew.

May we take the time to pause during the busyness of the day to reflect upon all we have. Compared to the majority of the world, we truly are fortunate, most fortunate. We do have hope. Most of all, we are privileged to be in a profession that can bring hope to others—physically, emotionally, and even spiritually.

Thank you for being "hope-givers" to those in need. In doing so, you are making a difference—one life at a time.

CHAPTER 55

La Esperanza

"Sh-h-h ninito, no llores. Dios te ama. Sh-h-h, little one, don't cry. God loves you." Over and over, I whispered these words to the frail Honduran boy as I gently stroked his thin, black hair. I guessed his age to be around 3 years, but his emaciated body made it difficult to know. So frail, so frightened, so alone—my heart ached to comfort him.

I had met him only an hour before. I was on a medical mission to the tiny town of La Esperanza, in the mountains west of Tegucigalpa. I was with a team of other providers and support staff to provide basic medical care to this most underserved part of Honduras. This was my fourth mission to Central America, and with every one, my heart was being broken.

Each mission was a catharsis for my soul, cleansing me of the built-up frustrations and pressures from years in clinical medicine. Not yet 50 years old, I was beginning to burn out. More and more, I questioned if I had made a mistake going into medicine. My heart was hardening, and my passion for medicine and my compassion for people were eroding. These mission trips allowed me to experience medicine in its purest form, unencumbered by paperwork, managed care, and an increasingly litigious society. I felt joy again in serving the people of Honduras, in simply serving and loving others.

Little did I know that God would use this little boy to minister to me.

As I was seeing patients each day, several women on the team saw the need for the children to be bathed, deloused, and dressed in clean clothes. They scoured the surrounding area and bought all the children's clothes and shoes they could find. Bathing stations using large trash cans were set up, and each child was washed, hair deloused, and new clothes and shoes provided. The laughter and delight of the children reverberated throughout the site. Word spread and more children came!

I wanted to be part of this. I decided to take half a day off from the clinic and spend the time helping wherever I could with the children.

He was the first I saw.

He cried incessantly, though weakly, his ebony eyes brimming with tears. His thin arms and legs were covered with dirt, too weak to resist the help we offered. As carefully as I could, I cleaned him. He left dressed in fresh, new clothes and shoes—no longer crying, but not smiling either.

An hour later, he was back. His new clothes were soiled, and a feeble cry was coming from trembling lips. As he stood before me, I carefully removed his clothes and shoes. I laid him down on the sun-drenched walkway and began cleaning him again.

Thoughts of my own boys, now nearly grown, rushed back, and I was overwhelmed with the need to show this little one the love and care that was missing from his life, a life of poverty compounded by physical and emotional neglect.

His crying continued, barely audible at times. He lay motionless, his head turned to the side, while he continued to stare as if looking for someone.

Suddenly, memories of rocking my boys as infants came flooding back. I began whispering a soft *sh-h-h* in his ear just as I had done with my sons, telling him again and again, "No llores, niñito, no llores. Dios te ama."

His soft sobs eased, and he looked at me with his ebony eyes. He calmly lay there as I finished cleaning him, all the while continuing to whisper to him as lovingly as I could. Once he was dressed, he was taken away, and I did not see him again.

In that brief moment in time with this Honduran boy, I was reminded of why I went into medicine - to serve others. The years of demanding work, long nights on call, administrative headaches, and managed care had slowly hardened my heart. God used this little one to begin a softening of my heart and a restoration of my soul.

CHAPTER 56

The Hands

The hands were heavily stained black, the skin marked with severe eczematous changes, yet she made no mention of them. She was a young mother who had come to the clinic to have her 6-month-old baby boy seen by the "doctors from America."

I was the team leader of a faith-based medical team serving on the outskirts of Nouakchott, the capital of Mauritania in Northwest Africa. We were there to provide primary medical care and public health teaching in support of a wonderful Swiss couple who ran a malnutrition clinic for the children of this impoverished country. Mostly, though, we came to love and serve.

Nouakchott sits on the edge of the vast Sahara Desert. The people we served had been primarily nomadic, as had their ancestors for centuries before them. They had been forced by an extended drought (who knew a drought could even occur in the Sahara!) to find another way to survive. The physical and emotional needs were as great as I have seen in 20 years of leading medical missions internationally.

I examined her baby and reassured her that he was healthy. My eyes, though, kept going back to her hands. Finally, I asked to see them. Painful fissures traversed the blackened skin. I asked about her work. She had two jobs, one washing dishes, the other dyeing cloth, her hands exposed daily to hours of hot water and caustic irritants. She had no gloves to protect them, no moisturizer to soothe and heal them. She simply did what she had to do to provide for her family.

She was typical of the Islamic women we saw that week. Her face was unseen, hidden by her *malafa*, a scarf wrapped over the head and covering the face, leaving only the eyes exposed. Her eyes were dark, intense, reflecting an inner strength and determination. I told her how much I respected her for being the strong woman and mother that she was. She sat up straight and looked at me, her eyes *smiling* back. She thanked me and stood to leave.

I wondered what would become of her and her baby. Did she have hope that her life would get better? I wanted to believe so. To live without hope is not to truly live.

The majority of people in the world live with no hope of things getting better. Every day is a struggle to survive. Each of you has seen this, too. It may be that a patient is facing a critical illness, grieving the heartbreak of loss, or experiencing the devastation of Alzheimer's. In the busyness of life, may you not miss *"the hands"* in front of you. May the needs of others become personal to you, as they become more real to you.

Thank you for seeing that need and going to it. In doing so, you bring hope and with hope, you bring life, and that makes all the difference.

CHAPTER 57

Back into the Mountains

She shook her head no, eyes brimming with tears, chin quivering with emotion. I told her again that without further care, her son would never have use of his arm and possibly could die. Her voice trembling, she told me her husband would beat her if she returned home without the boy.

She placed her son on their horse, his newly bandaged arm in a makeshift sling. I gave her antibiotics and medicine for pain, still pleading to let us take him to the nearest hospital. Shaking her head again, she turned and led the horse back into the mountains of central Honduras, the boy silent, staring back at me, the contrast between his tiny body and the horse striking.

Only an hour earlier, they had arrived at our clinic. She had heard an American medical team had arrived for the week, and she desperately wanted her son to be seen. The day before, while he was cutting bamboo with a machete, a mis-swing cut into his left forearm. She had bandaged it with cloth as best she could and made the several-hour trip by horseback to see us.

I was amazed how stoic he was at only 8 years of age, his toughness forged by the circumstances of his life. No tears, no sound, his ebony eyes watching my every move. I removed the blood-caked bandage, revealing a gaping wound traversing his left forearm, exposed muscles appearing to be completely cut through. Remarkably, the main arteries were intact.

A nurse cleaned the wound, and then I began to carefully explore the extent of damage. He needed urgent surgical attention to save his arm and possibly his life. The nearest hospital was several hours away.

My host partner, Ricardo, began calling. In a matter of minutes, a physician, a friend of Ricardo 's-was on the phone. IV fluids and antibiotics were started, a sterile dressing carefully applied. In less than an hour, he was ready to go by car.

I explained to the mother all we had done and the arrangements we had fortunately been able to make. Without our intervention, he would have been refused care at any hospital because of her inability to pay. This is an all-too-common scenario in many countries—no money, no care.

I was anticipating tears of joy and gratitude. Instead came the sideways shake of her head and the flowing of tears.

I have led over 40 medical missions to countries in Central America, Eastern Europe, Central Asia, and Northwest Africa, experiencing their unique beauty and the richness of their vastly different cultures. I have also seen the desperate poverty and ever-present hopelessness with which the people live.

We are most fortunate to live where we do, without the daily struggles to survive that are common to so many in the world.

The eyes of that little boy are always a reminder of that to me.

CHAPTER 58

Broken by a Smile

As I have led medical missions internationally, there often occurs an event that becomes etched in my mind, and I cannot forget. This happened most recently in Mauritania, located in Northwest Africa. We were there to support a nutrition center run by two Swiss missionaries in the capital city of Nouakchott. The center cared for severely malnourished children. It was heartbreaking to see these children clinging to life.

Significant poverty created by a "spider web" of causes is common in this part of the world, literally surrounded by the Sahara Desert. The beauty of the Sahara at sunrise was quite a contrast to the prevalent desperation and hopelessness that permeated everything. Yet, out of this came a reminder that something good, even beautiful, can be found.

That something was a smile.

A smile from two children, and it broke me.

Mauritania was my first time serving in a Muslim country. I admit to having some trepidation, but that quickly dissolved as I saw how appreciative, kind, and accepting the people were. The poverty, the need, and the hardships they faced daily quickly became apparent as the days went by.

The children, though, stole my heart. Despite the difficulties of their lives, they, like the countless children I have seen all over the world, were still happy. Life had not broken their spirits yet. Time would change that soon enough.

The two children, a brother and a sister, came to the clinic with their mother. She was dressed in the traditional *malafa*, with only a small portion of her face showing. I was immediately struck by how thin and dirty they were. Neither child smiled nor looked at me. They were too afraid, and as I found out later, I was the first "white person" they had ever seen.

I quickly began doing all I could to get them to relax. Simple "smiley face" stickers did it!

I placed one on the back of each child's hand, and you would have thought I had given them their dream present! Their eyes opened wide and both broke into big smiles, showing teeth in need of much repair but still joyous all the same.

I had a picture taken with them to remember that moment, a moment when my heart was broken by a smile. In this case, two smiles. Even in the face of great need, children can be happy.

I write this story to ask: When was the last time you allowed yourself to be "broken by a smile", be it from a child, a grateful patient, or an appreciative family member?

When was the last time you let your guard down, put your busyness aside, and let a smile remind you of how fortunate you are to do what you do?

What you do, only a few are privileged to do. We all need to be reminded, for it is all too easy to forget in today's world of medicine.

Let your heart be broken by a smile. You'll be glad you did.

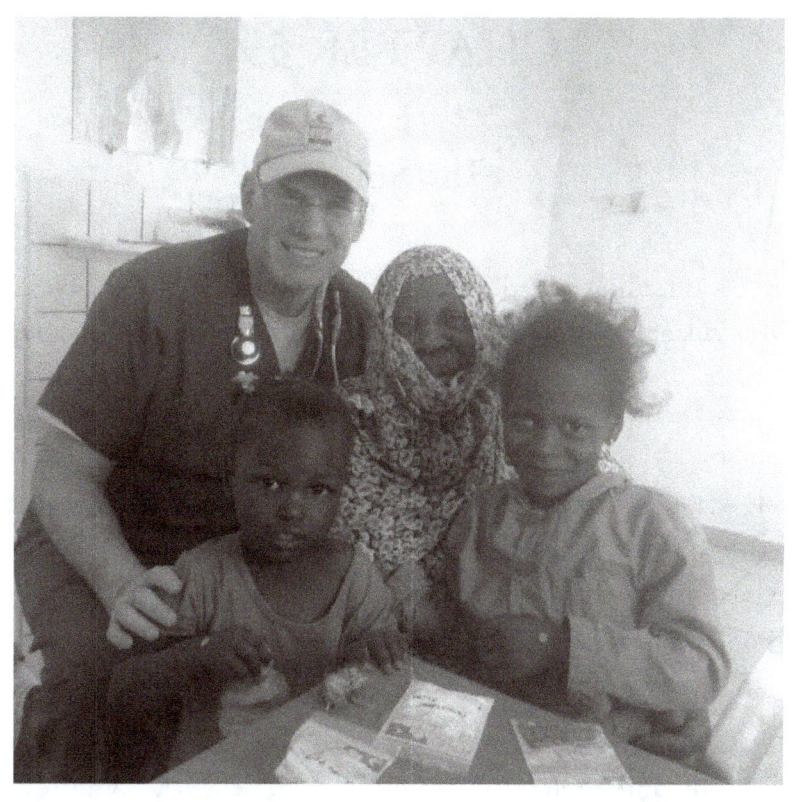

CHAPTER 59

The Smile

I was leading a medical team in Moldova. We were serving in a village of around 5,000, with its dirt roads, small stone houses, and where indoor plumbing was a "city" thing. The clinic we ran had just finished for the day. My interpreter and I had seen at least 50 patients, and we were exhausted. That's when I first saw him. He was standing at the door to the clinic—a gangly teenager dressed in a white shirt and black pants. The look on his face, the way he stood with slumped shoulders, arms at his side, eyes downcast—all cried out: "Help me!"

I found myself irritated that he had "suddenly" shown up. I told my interpreter to tell him to come back tomorrow morning. Her eyes locked on mine, and she said, "We have to see him. He needs our help. Don't you see that?" She was right. We were there to love and serve in any way we could.

I motioned him in, and he slowly walked toward us, head down. He made me think of the village dogs that roamed the streets, neglected, beaten, starving, their tails between their legs. What was his story?

In my many years of leading medical missions, I have learned that the emotional needs of those we serve are often as great as the physical. This is especially true in Moldova, a country without hope, after centuries of oppression, wars, and

160

nearly 100 years of Soviet rule. A corrupt government, a crumbling economy, and high unemployment have forced many a mother, father, or both to leave their children with friends or family to find work in a neighboring country. It was the only way they could survive.

A Moldovan pastor once told me, *"The world has either never heard of Moldova—or it doesn't care."*

Through my interpreter, I asked if he was having any physical problems. He shook his head no, eyes fixed on his hands. I then asked how things were at home. He began to cry. His father was an alcoholic, as were most men in the village. When drunk, he became violent and beat his mother and himself. He had heard from others who had been to our clinic that "the Americans" were kind, compassionate, and spoke of a loving God. He had no place else to go. So, he came to us.

I reached my hands out to him. He gripped them tightly as my interpreter spoke of God's love, with a compassion and caring he had never experienced. His entire demeanor began to change. He listened intently, eyes now focused on us. We told him about the Moldovan pastor who had invited us to serve in the village, and asked if he would be willing to meet him. He immediately nodded yes.

We stood up, and wrapping my arms around him, I prayed for him. He thanked us and turned to leave. When he reached the door, he turned and looked at us. I hardly recognized him as the same person who had appeared so suddenly less than an hour before. Then he smiled. Not a faint smile—a big smile. He waved one last time and left. I will never forget "the smile".

It is a reminder of the difference a person can make in the lives of others.

May each of you have your own "reminder" of the difference you make in the lives of those you serve. This is where the human side of medicine happens and the joy that comes with it.

We are better people and physicians for having experienced it.

CHAPTER 60

The Mother

"Andy, we need you. Now!"

These words are common to hear as a team leader of medical missions. I have served in some of the poorest countries, where there is little or no access to medical care. You never knew what emergency would suddenly appear at the clinic.

This one I would not forget. It was hot and equally humid in the tiny Honduran village. The human need was great. Hundreds came daily by any means possible, foot, horseback, mule, oxen, motorbike—often traveling many hours to be seen. Each succeeding day grew busier as word of our presence spread.

The people, as always, were loving, appreciative, and thankful.

She was in her 20s, the mother of four. Her last baby had been born the day before. However, later that night, she developed a fever and abdominal pain. Within hours, she rapidly deteriorated. The nearest hospital was a day's walk because she lived deep in the mountains. Late that night, her husband and five other men placed her on a blanket and began a six-hour journey over treacherous mountain trails to reach the American doctors they had heard about.

Septic, in fulminant pulmonary edema, she was seizing every few minutes. IV fluids and antibiotics were started, an oral airway placed, and, remembering a long-ago intervention for pulmonary edema, I began rotating tourniquets. We had no IV Lasix, no endotracheal tube, no Ambu bag, no oxygen. The lack of basic infrastructure and the logistics of carrying our medicines, supplies, and equipment with us from the States limit what we can bring and do.

There was a small hospital an hour away. The local pastor called for an "ambulance." On arrival, I opened the rear doors to find a shell of an ambulance. We lifted her into the back, while Wendy, a third-year medical student, and I climbed in beside her. She began vomiting between seizures. We continued rotating tourniquets and clearing her airway as her lungs filled further with fluid. The temperature inside was well over 100°F. We struggled in the suffocating heat—no air conditioning, no windows to open, and the smell of vomitus permeating the air.

We prayed. On arrival, she was immediately taken to the OR, where a D&C was performed.

She died a few hours later.

To most of the world, you and I live and work in "paradise." May this story be a reminder of how fortunate we are, and what a privilege it is to do what we do. Most of all, though, I am thankful for you.

CHAPTER 61

Doing Small Things with Great Love

"Why do I do what I do?" This is a question I'm sure many of you have asked yourself at one time or another. Who hasn't been asked the question, "Why did you become a doctor?" Obviously, I can't answer for you, but I can for myself, and my answer, hopefully, will resonate with many of you.

Years ago, when there were no limits on work hours in residency, when hospital call meant 36-hour stretches without sleep, and when only a "wimp" called their attending in the middle of the night, I would have answered this question much differently than I do now.

I would have said:

"I want to help people."

"I like challenging things."

"I enjoy learning new things."

"I want to make a good living."

There's nothing wrong with those answers.

But as the years went by, medicine began to change. The patients were older, sicker, more complicated, with more technology needed to care for them. I found myself working harder and longer, seeing more patients just to maintain the status quo.

Those answers were no longer enough to keep me going. I began to question why I did what I did.

My answers had become shallow. Superficial.

Then I did my first medical mission to Guatemala in 2000, and my life irreversibly changed. I'm not saying you need to be doing a mission trip. I am simply saying that for me, this was the catalyst that changed my answer to that question.

What was that answer? It was the simple realization that I wanted to make a difference, whether in the life of one person, many people, or something much bigger.

The desire to make a difference, I believe, is innate to us in one degree or another. What does that look like?

For me, it was making a difference one life at a time. That one person can, in turn, make a difference in the lives of others, in ways we may never know.

I love the old African saying:

"If you think you're too small to make a difference, try spending the night in a closed room with a mosquito!"

More powerfully, I love the quote from Mother Teresa:

"We can do no great things, only small things with great love."

There are people who have done truly great things. But most of us do "only small things."

It is how we do the small things that makes a difference: To love and serve others. To bring hope where there is no hope.

And when all else fails medically, to simply be there for that person.

To hold them. To sit with them. Even to cry with them.

In the busyness and hard work of medicine, these may seem insignificant.

But they are not. They can sustain you when the answers of the past no longer do.

You make a difference to each of our patients, and for that, I thank you.

CHAPTER 62

The Girl

She sat across from me, a Soviet-era wooden table between us. I was leading a medical mission to a village in Moldova. Once part of the Soviet Union, Moldova struggled to survive as an independent country. For many, to live in Moldova is to live with little hope of anything ever getting better.

The young people are most affected by the collapse of the Soviet Union. They have few job opportunities. They cannot travel freely except to a few "approved" countries. They are prisoners in their own country.

As a Moldovan pastor once told me, *"The world either has never heard of Moldova, or does not care about us."*

She was unsmiling, eyes downcast, shoulders drooping. At 15 years of age, she had the striking features so typical of Eastern European women. Through my interpreter, I asked the usual questions as I took her history. In a barely audible voice, never looking up at me, she spoke of having abdominal pain off and on for the past several months. Further questioning revealed no other worrisome symptoms.

I reassured her, gave her some vitamins, and spoke to her about why we were there as a medical team. After praying with her, she quietly thanked me and left without another word. Not long afterward, she was back. This time complaining of chronic, recurrent headaches.

I was surprised she returned, but I didn't give it too much thought. I addressed her concerns, reassured her, and sent her on her way. As I was seeing the next patient, I could see her standing to the side, looking at me with what? Sadness? Hopelessness? Desperation?

At first, I was irritated. Had I not already seen her twice? Could she not see that I was busy and that there were many other patients? But she continued to stand; waiting, watching.

It was then I realized there was something more going on than I had realized.

This was a cry for help.

I called her over and asked if there was anything further I could do for her. She became anxious, glancing nervously around the room—as if looking for something, or someone. She brought up a new physical complaint, and again I reassured her.

"How are things at home?" I asked. Where did she live? Did she live with her parents? Was anything going on that she needed to talk about? My gut told me something was very wrong. After all, Moldova is the central hub of human trafficking in Europe.

Was she trapped in that most horrible of situations?

With compassion and care, my interpreter translated my questions. Her chin began to quiver.

The tears began to flow. She nodded her head yes—softly saying that her older brother was sexually abusing her, and had been for over two years.

They lived with their grandparents, as their parents were both working out of country—as is very common in Moldova. Financially, it was the only way many families could survive. The grandparents knew nothing. She was too afraid and ashamed to speak up. Her brother would beat her if she did.

My heart broke for her as I fully comprehended her situation—and the fear she lived with every day.

Whether human trafficking or domestic violence, the trauma, the pain, the guilt, the shame, the hopelessness—are ever present. She could not return to that environment.

I spoke to the local pastor and explained the situation. He would have his wife take her into their home and get her the help she needed. It would be a long road to recovery for her. I do not know what happened to her after we left.

There is always the realization that this is all too common a situation. How often do we miss the subtle cries for help, because we are too busy to hear?

We live in a hurting world. People are not always "fine" as they say when you ask the proverbial question, *"How are you?"*

Too often, they are not fine. Or good. Or wonderful. It is easier to say so than to admit the painful reality in which they live.

We are often allowed into the most intimate aspects of a patient's life, the good and the bad.

The sacredness of this relationship is a special privilege.

How often do we miss a cry for help?

Medicine is much more than the medical care we provide. There is also an emotional, physical, and spiritual component, caring for the whole person.

To do so, we must be ready to see the need in front of us. Otherwise, we will miss it. There is too much at stake. People are crying for our help. Are you hearing them?

CHAPTER 63

A Knock at the Door

"There will be a knock at the door," says Rene, an El Salvadoran pastor and my close friend, "and they will say, '*Give us your daughter or we will kill you and your family.*'"

He continues, "Gangs control many of the villages. They are in the schools; they are in this school! If the leader sees a girl that he likes, no matter her age, he sends members of his gang to her home and demands that she be given to them, to be used however the leader decides. If the parents refuse, the gang members keep their word and take the girl anyway. When a boy reaches the age of 10, if he does not join a gang, he may be killed. This is one reason why many of the children arriving at the U.S. borders are alone, without parents or a significant other. Their parents had to make a decision—a decision of life or death. A last resort. A gut-wrenching decision. Yet the decision becomes all too clear: it is safer for their children to make this most perilous journey than to remain in their own home."

I listen in disbelief as I sit on the crumbling concrete steps of the village school where our medical clinic is temporarily located for the week. The village lies on the side of an inactive, waterless volcano, where large cisterns dot the mountainside, collecting precious rainwater for the people's everyday needs.

This is my 12th year leading medical teams to a country and a people I have come to love deeply. It has become my *segunda casa*, my second home. Yet somehow, I had not heard this story, the brutal, lived reality for so many in El Salvador.

It is a beautiful country of volcanic mountains and rock-strewn beaches. Its natural beauty stands in stark contrast to the ever-present violence and intimidation of the gangs. Even the capital, San Salvador, cannot escape this dark reality.

Mara Salvatrucha.

MS-13.

These are names that elicit fear in every El Salvadoran. Most of all, the fear of a knock at the door.

Often, "Coyotes" will take these children—and others willing to sacrifice everything for a chance at a life with a glimmer of hope—on this most hazardous trek, where illness, injury, and death are ever present. They are soulless mercenaries who feed on and live off this agonizing reality, extracting a precious cost from desperate families. A cost of money, of fractured families, and of lives.

To live without hope is not to live. It is simply to exist. So the decision is made. The children are sent. Hope for a better life for them, and for the loved ones left behind, becomes the powerful driving force.

In the villages, lacking many of the modern luxuries of larger towns and cities, little is known about the news of the world. Life is a daily struggle for survival.

They know nothing of the "immigration problem" that is often front-page news in the U.S.

They are oblivious to the polarizing issue it has become in our country, with all its ugly faces.

They only know what they've always heard: That America stands for freedom. Opportunity. And most of all, hope. They want that for themselves, but especially for their children.

So this heart-wrenching story is repeated over and over again. And the tears fall. Hearts break.
And families are separated.

Many in the U.S. ask the question: "Why?" Why would parents send their children on a potential death march? How could they ever do that? How could they be so heartless, unloving, irresponsible?

Did they not care for their children, love their children?

"I would never do that," we all too easily say, without hesitation.

But in those same circumstances… would we?

Fortunately, we do not live in such a cruel reality. My heart aches. My eyes glisten. There are children at the school now—children we will see in the clinic—who live in this *Twilight Zone* of reality.
I feel helpless.

As a physician, I seek to comfort, treat, and heal. As a father, I do everything I can to love and protect my children.

The people of El Salvador seek to do the same for those they love. No matter the cost. No matter the sacrifice. May we not forget this. I never will.

CHAPTER 64

Your Greatest Gift

I stood inside the door of *una choza*, Spanish for "a hut". The walls were bamboo and sunbaked mud; the floor, broom-swept dirt. Two open windows were partially covered by tattered cloth. There was no running water, no electricity. The acrid smell of smoke from the wood fire in the open brick oven permeated the air.

Then I saw her.

Lying on a bed made of wood and rope was a young woman. To my astonishment, she had a gastric feeding tube and a Foley catheter. Her arms and legs were atrophied, contracted. Her breathing was shallow and rapid. Rivulets of sweat traced down her face—the oppressive heat and humidity of Honduras in August punctuating the surreal scene in front of me.

Wendy, a third-year medical student, and I were doing home visits as part of a medical team serving in El Triunfo, a village of 5,000 people in southern Honduras. We traveled by truck over rock-strewn, dirt roads, crossing several small streams to reach a remote village of about 50 families. We didn't know what kind of patient we'd be seeing. Most often, the home visits were to see the elderly, bedridden by severe arthritis or a debilitating stroke. But not this time.

She was 21 and had been healthy until the year before, when she suddenly collapsed, never to regain consciousness. Her family had carried her in the back of a truck, over mountainous terrain and rough roads, to the hospital in Tegucigalpa, an 8-hour journey.

There, they received the news: nothing more could be done.

Their hopes shattered, she returned home in the same way she had arrived—this time with a permanent feeding tube and Foley catheter.

To my surprise, her husband handed me a CT scan of her head, done at the hospital. I raised the films to the sunlight. A large intracerebral bleed was readily apparent. I slowly lowered the telltale images and looked at Wendy. Her past history was now painfully clear.

Clinically, she was infected. She had a fever. Her urine was concentrated and cloudy, a recent change, according to her husband. I told him we had antibiotics we could administer through the feeding tube, and I explained the importance of keeping her well hydrated.

As we prepared to leave, our hearts heavy, her husband began asking more questions. Could we not give her something to make her well again?

And then I understood.

He believed that, as a doctor from the United States, I could heal her. That I would bring her back to him. After all, I was from America, and America had the best of everything.

Such unrealistic expectations are not uncommon.

I explained what the CT scan showed and confirmed that there was nothing I, nor anyone else, could do. She would not recover.

He began to sob—head lowered, hands covering his face—as all remaining hope vanished. We took his hands in ours, sat with him, and prayed.

What else could we do?

You know this pain. The heartbreak. The suffering. It is part of being a physician. It is part of life.

Thinking back on the 30 years I practiced Internal Medicine, I remember best the patients for whom everything medically possible was done, only to fail. In their moments of deepest despair, all I could do was be present. Hold their hand. Listen to them. Cry with them.

Words are not always necessary. As physicians, we want to heal our patients when possible. But maybe, just maybe, our greatest gift to a patient is not healing, because healing is transient.

Maybe, instead, your greatest gift is your ability to be completely present with a patient's suffering—allowing it to transform you, and in doing so, to transform it for them as well.

Your presence becomes everything to the patient who feels they are losing everything.

As you face what your patient faces, you are better able to bring compassion to them, and maybe, I believe, better able to extend that same compassion to yourself, as you continue the hard work of medicine.

Thank you for your selfless service to those in their darkest time of despair.

CHAPTER 65

Making A Difference

I was somewhere over the Atlantic Ocean, heading to Ukraine "to make a difference", or so I hoped. I was leading a medical mission to this beautiful yet poor and war-torn country. I was watching the movie *First Man* about the landing of Apollo 11 on the moon, that epic day in July 1969. I was not quite 14 years of age at that time, but I vividly remember the live, grainy TV footage of that first step by Neil Armstrong. Millions across the world watched, breath held, as he did so. This was the culmination of over a decade of meticulous preparation and selfless dedication to a goal, a dream, far bigger than anything ever done before. It began with the first Mercury space launch, then the Gemini series, and finally the Apollo missions to realize what President Kennedy had promised in 1962: before the decade was over, to put a man on the moon and bring him safely back.

Throughout my elementary school years in the '60s, teachers would stop classwork and turn on the generic black-and-white TV so we could watch the live launches of every "next step" toward that seemingly impossible goal.

I was inspired—inspired by the sacrifice, courage, and perseverance of Neil Armstrong, by every individual who had risked their life, by those who had lost theirs, and by the families who endured, so that "one small step for man" would become a "giant leap for mankind". I tried to hide the tears in the darkness of the plane. Memories from that time suddenly surfaced—a time when my future was before me, unknown, waiting to be discovered, explored, and experienced.

It caused me to posit, "Have I made a difference with my life? Have I lived a life that counted? Must I do something truly *great* to make a difference?" Up until I saw the movie, I would have answered unequivocally yes—that I had made a difference and was still making a difference. However, after watching it, I was not so sure anymore. What does it look like to make a difference, to live a life that counts? Do you have to be a Neil Armstrong, a Mother Teresa, a Martin Luther King, an Abraham Lincoln, or a Mahatma Gandhi?

Leading medical missions, I have learned that every one of us makes a difference, and it *can* be significant. We do it "one life at a time". Every surgery, every medical intervention, every restored bit of health, every loving touch, kind word, listening ear, and "stained glass heart" makes a difference in someone's life. This is what you do every day, yet it is so easy to lose sight of that in the world that is medicine today.

You may never know the full impact you've had on the lives of those you've touched, but there *will* be an impact and a ripple effect.

Thank you for being a difference-maker. Thank you for the years of sacrifice you made so you could make a difference in the lives you touch. You are living a life that counts, and I, for one, am grateful for you.

SECTION IV
STORIES

CHAPTER 66

Playing Catch

The baseball hissed as it sped toward me, followed by a loud *pop* as I caught it in the pocket of my Wilson A2000 baseball glove, a glove I never thought I would own. In 1969, at $50, it was far too expensive for my parents. I was 14, and baseball was my identity, my significance, my reason for being, my worldview as seen through the eyes of a boy living in a world of non-sameness, a world in which the only dependable constants revolved around baseball. I was an "Army Brat".

My father was a career Army officer. I attended 10 different schools in 12 years. Friends were hard to make for my older brother, Michael, and me, as we learned early that civilian kids were not very accepting of "outsiders." Sports broke down the door of "them versus us". Without sports, especially baseball, I'm not sure how I would have navigated the life that was mine at the time.

Christmas 1969 was a most memorable one. Each present carried the potential to be *the one*—the A2000. My youthful excitement and hope quickly met a cruel reality. As I looked over my now-opened presents, trying to hide my disappointment, my father, almost as if scripted from the iconic movie *A Christmas Story*, said, "Andy, what is that behind the chair by the tree?" My heart pounded as I retrieved the "missed" present. I tore away the wrapping, and there it was. *THE GLOVE*. Wilson A2000, engraved in the reddish-brown leather for all to see! I buried my face in the pocket of the glove, inhaling deeply, letting the richness and earthiness of leather fill my nostrils. I pounded my fist into the pocket, reveling in the feel and sound that were synonymous with baseball.

I went to the kitchen and retrieved the large blue Crisco can filled with white lard that my mother always had for cooking. I began applying it, first to the pocket and inside webbing of the glove, then the remainder on the outside. The leather darkened, softened, as I prepared this extension of my left hand for the play ahead.

Always, in early spring, as the weather warms, the flowers bloom, and the grass greens, the memories of baseball come flooding back. The excitement and anticipation before a game were almost as intense as Christmas Eve! I would put on my uniform hours before the game, making sure the white sanitary hose, pro-cut stockings, and gig line were perfectly adjusted. Then followed an interminable pacing back and forth, asking my mother over and over, "Is it time yet to leave for the game?"

The joy I felt upon taking the field; my cleats gripping the red dirt; the scent of freshly cut grass enveloping me; the sweat, dirt, and dank smell of the below-ground dugout, bubblegum wrappers and paper snow cone cups scattered about the floor; the click of metal cleats, "real baseball shoes", on a hard surface once I had graduated to playing with the "big boys"; hitting a baseball on the sweet spot of my Harmon Killebrew–engraved Louisville Slugger; the sting in my glove hand from a hard-thrown ball.

But the memories I cherish most are of playing catch with my father. He was my bigger-than-life hero. Even now, I can see him with the ball in hand—tall, strong, his muscular arms and chest the envy of all my friends. Three years of my childhood, he was away, including two combat tours in Vietnam. But when he was home, he was fully present. I savored every catch, every throw, every moment.

I cannot watch the movie *Field of Dreams* without crying when Kevin Costner looks at his father and says those magical words, *"Dad, want to play catch?"*

It's so easy, when you're young, to wish time away as you chase a goal you believe will make your life complete and happy. In doing so, we fail to appreciate those special moments—moments we *should* be cherishing. Time is a blur until, suddenly, one day, it's no longer a blur. Instead, it becomes a motion picture in slow motion, each frame a reminder of a moment in time that should have been savored... only to be lost in our quest for what?

Thank you, Daddy, for the memories you gave me. I miss you.

CHAPTER 67

The Man in the Red Sash

July 2, 1973, a day etched forever in my mind. A day I remember as if it happened yesterday, even though 50 years have passed. A day I thought would never come and then, when it did, would never end. It was the day I entered West Point as a 17-year-old kid with big dreams to "become an Airborne, Ranger, Infantryman and lead men in combat." That was my goal in life at that time.

My life changed the moment I reported to the "Man in the Red Sash," a senior cadet responsible for the training of the 1,400 new cadets entering that day with me. Of those, 697 of us graduated four years later.

That hot July day began my journey to becoming a man. The change started immediately. I reported to that senior cadet who, to me, seemed bigger than life, all-powerful and all-knowing. In many ways, he and the other First-Class men (as seniors at West Point are called) were. After all, they had survived their first year and the two that followed. They had only one more year left, and then they were free. I vividly remember thinking that my graduation would never come. Four years felt like an eternity to a 17-year-old who, at that moment, wasn't sure he could make it through the day, much less the two months of intense training that would follow. Those two months were appropriately called "Beast Barracks," and I soon found out why.

185

"Beast Barracks" existed to begin the transformation from civilian to soldier, as well as to instill the customs and traditions of West Point. Talk about change — this was change with a capital "C". It had another purpose as well: to identify and eliminate any new cadet who did not have what it took to succeed at West Point and become an officer in the U.S. Army. To succeed meant being mentally, emotionally, and physically tough enough to withstand the rigors of West Point. If one could not handle these artificially imposed pressures, then how could they be expected to hold up under the most extreme of mental and physical duress — combat?

Those months epitomized change in every way possible. I endured sleep deprivation, food denial (a very common practice at the time), rigorous physical conditioning, hard military training, and verbal and emotional abuse from the seniors training us. In addition, I had to memorize massive amounts of "Plebe Knowledge" required of every new cadet. This information was contained in a small book we all received that first day called *Bugle Notes*. Now you know where the name came from! I lost 12 pounds that summer, and I didn't have 12 pounds to lose.

During this time of dramatic change, I was learning much about myself, about others, and about what it meant to be part of a team. Teamwork, unity, and togetherness were drilled into us until they became a part of who we were. Expressions such as "cooperate and graduate," "help your buddy," "no one left behind," and my class motto, "Esprit de Corps," were ever present. No one successfully completes four years at West Point alone. If you do not learn how to work with others as a team, you will not make it through.

Those four years were hard work with very little play, though when we played, we played hard. Much sacrifice was required, and when I graduated and drove through those gates that last time on June 8, 1977, I was not sure whether what I had been through had been worth the emotional, mental, and physical trials I faced. I actually flipped up my rearview mirror so I would not see even a glimpse of West Point behind me.

Much change had occurred during those four years, and I was not convinced all of it was good. As the years passed, the bad memories began to fade and were replaced by better ones. Doors opened up for me that I am convinced never would have opened without my education and training there. I eventually realized those four years had been worth it.

Why do I tell you this story? Just as I went through changes that affected my life in ways I could never have imagined, each of you has gone through times of change, and continue to do so. Your own extensive medical training and life experiences have created these changes — for the good, mostly, but at times for the not-so-good. Each of you has become an expert in change.

No matter the change, no matter the challenges ahead, you keep moving forward because that is what you do; adapt and persevere. The ability to adapt and persevere has helped make you who you are today. Is change easy? No, but it is critical if we are to fulfill our calling to help and serve others.

Thank you for being that person. Thank you for the sacrifices you have made and continue to make so that our patients can receive the best care.

CHAPTER 68

Stories from My Father

I am sitting in a hospital room in Birmingham, Alabama. My 87-year-old father lies in a Hill-Rom bed, frail, thin, and weak. This once physically strong and imposing man is a shell of who he was, of who he will always be in my mind, a larger-than-life Airborne, Ranger, Infantry officer. A man who served two combat tours in Vietnam, my hero. I, too, wanted to be like him. That is why I chose to go to West Point. My father is the single most influential person in my life.

The "naturalness" of his dying is slowly progressing. I understand this. It is very hard to watch, and I can do nothing about it. He cannot walk. He cannot even stand alone with a four-point walker. He can no longer do the 100 push-ups and 100 bar dips that were his daily norm until the age of 80. The façade of immortality is gone.

My heart breaks, and I grieve.

He grieves as well. The realization that he may never walk again, nor return to his home, work on his beloved cars, or build another remote-control plane, is beginning to set in. What can you say and do in times like this? As the only doctor in the family, they look to me for answers to questions and help with decisions. At times, I feel resentful, as I want to be his son, not his doctor. But most of the time, I am grateful I can help.

Out of this comes an unexpected blessing, an opportunity to have a special one-on-one time with him. We talk about anything and everything. I learned things about him I never knew. He spoke of the hardships growing up in the Great Depression, of how, as a five-year-old, he would walk five miles to the nearby airport to watch the biplanes take off and land. Occasionally, he would be paid five cents to sweep the hangar floors. With that, he would buy a Coke and "nurse" it throughout the day. If he was really lucky, he could get a Moon Pie with it.

He talked about how his mother would make fruitcakes in September, wrap them in cheesecloth, and keep them on top of the icebox until Christmas. To this day, he loves fruitcake.

What surprised me most was how close I came to losing my father in combat during his two tours in Vietnam. God's protection was readily apparent. I sat there amazed, humbled, and thankful.

Sadly, it often takes an unpleasant event to bring people together so these stories can be shared.

As physicians, patients will reach out to us in their time of grief, pain, or fear. They, too, need someone to hear their stories. We become that someone, and in doing so, we acknowledge their humanity. We ultimately become their storytellers, and they become a part of who we are as a person, as a human being, who one day will face our own mortality and need someone to listen to our stories.

CHAPTER 69

A Serious Business

He stood silently, his eyes fixed on us, immaculately dressed in a dark three-piece suit adorned with a gold watch and chain. His hair was meticulously groomed, a brightly colored bow tie centered perfectly on a freshly starched white shirt, wire collar stays in place, black wing-tip shoes glistening. Gold cufflinks and military-like, sharply creased pants, with just a subtle break of the cuff on the shoe tops, completed the picture. He could have passed any inspection I went through at West Point. Then he spoke:

"Medicine is a serious business," he said firmly. "You should never smile, joke, or laugh with a patient, nor sit on a patient's bed. At all times, you must be professional and maintain a proper distance physically and emotionally. You must not allow yourself to become emotionally affected by a patient's condition, no matter how bad it may be. Otherwise, you risk losing your authority and your objectivity, which could end up harming the patient."

He was my instructor in history and physical examination during my second year at the University of Alabama School of Medicine in Birmingham. I was excited, as were my classmates, to take those first baby steps toward becoming a "real" doctor. His words burst that bubble of innocence. Speechless, we stood there, heads nodding dutifully, obediently, in unison. How could we respond otherwise, and what right did we have to say anything? He was, after all, a world-renowned cardiologist. We quickly understood our proper place in this intimidating new world of medicine in 1980.

I looked at him, in all his "glorious perfection," and thought, "This guy is full of crap. That's one of the most ridiculous things I've ever heard." Only a few years out of West Point and having served three years in Germany as an Army officer, I had heard my share of "wisdom" from those above me. Most of the time, I learned from it. But sometimes... well, this was a sometimes.

Of course, we all did exactly what he said during those weeks under his omnipotent, omniscient presence. He was hard on us, too. We learned how to do a complete history and physical exam to his demanding satisfaction. We memorized every review-of-systems question, reciting them back to him again and again. I was grateful for the high expectations he placed on us. We learned well.

However, I knew that as soon as I was on my own, caring for patients, I would be smiling, laughing, joking, and, heaven forbid, sitting on the side of their bed, as long as I knew it was okay with them. Being professional was not the issue.

For 30 years as an internist, I did just that. I believe patients do not care how much you know until they know how much you care. All people have an innate need to feel loved, cared for, and treated as persons of worth and value. This is especially true when they are most frightened, vulnerable, and dependent, as during illness or injury. This forms the foundation of the "sacred trust" that is the doctor-patient relationship.

This trust only happens when compassion, caring, empathy, and the warmth of love are both given and received. This is the "art of medicine" in its truest form. From trust springs hope. To live without hope is a terrible thing. The emotional pain of despair will soon follow. I know. I have experienced it both in the world and at the deepest level personally.

The world needs more hope-givers. Be that person. In doing so, the joy you once had, you can have again. Medicine is a serious business, but more importantly, it is a deeply personal, fully human endeavor. Humility, empathy, compassion, caring, and love are its fickle guardians.

The busyness and business of medicine can easily blind you to this truth. We build walls and wear masks as protection from the heartbreak, the loss, the hurt, the pain that surely will come. May you take down your wall, remove your mask, and let people see who you really are: a person, a physician who cares, understands, and is completely present with them no matter the circumstances.

Yes, medicine is a serious business, but far more than that, it is a privilege; albeit a hard one. Every day, what you do is important and makes a difference in the lives of those you touch.

Thank you for being that person.

CHAPTER 70

"Never!"

"Never! Never have I heard such words come from the mouth of a man!" Her right fist slammed the wooden tabletop. "I want to read that book right now!" She looked at Lloyd as if she had suddenly realized something precious had been kept from her.

We were in Moldova, the poorest country in Europe. Once part of the mighty Soviet Union, it was now an independent country struggling to navigate the dramatic upheaval caused by its collapse and the sudden newfound freedom. The road was difficult, as 100 years of corruption at every level of government proved nearly impossible to overcome. For the Moldovan people, their daily lives had not noticeably changed since the fall of Soviet hegemony. Hopelessness and despair remained, ever-present, like a heavy fog on a cold, drizzly morning, swallowing them whole. Communism or democracy, what did it matter?

Unemployment was rampant. Families were separated as husbands and wives, mothers and fathers, desperately sought work in neighboring countries, leaving their children with family or friends. Alcoholism was epidemic among men, fueled by culture and inflamed by despair. Moldova had become the central hub of human trafficking for Europe. It was the "worst hard times." As one Moldovan was heard to say, "The world has either forgotten Moldova or has never heard of it."

Lloyd and I were the team leaders of a faith-based medical mission. We had led other missions to Moldova and knew the culture, as well as the physical, emotional, and spiritual needs that permeated the country. The Russian Orthodox Church and atheism dominated the faith worldview. The concept of a loving, grace-filled, compassionate, and accessible God was foreign to them. The priests controlled all matters of faith, and more.

The Moldovan people lived a life where "The only end to pain is the graveyard," as an elderly, arthritis-crippled woman once said to me while we sat on the steps of her tiny cinder block home, devoid of running water and electricity. She had no hope of anything ever getting better.

Team members stay with host families in the village where we serve. This provides a uniquely wonderful opportunity to experience the culture and life of the people we are serving. The interpreters stay with us as well, allowing us to get to know them even better. Our interpreter was Peter, and he proved to be a rich source of cultural and historical knowledge, as well as our biggest encourager. Years later, we remain close friends.

The Wednesday night of our week in the village is spent with the host family as we share food, drink, and conversation. It is a wonderful time to better understand the lives they lead and their beliefs.

Our hosts were in their 50s. They were hardworking, tough, and resilient. Life gave them no other choice. They rarely smiled and identified as atheists.

194

After dinner, we sat in the living room and began asking questions about their lives, hoping to gain their trust. For the next two hours, we talked while they sat quietly, listening. Then, to our surprise, the husband began asking the hard questions about God and faith: His existence, good versus evil, creation versus evolution, and more.

We answered the ones we could, and when we could not, we spoke of faith. They began to relax and even smile. This gave Lloyd the opportunity to speak on a topic he is passionate about: how men are to love and serve their wives as Christ did the Church.

While he was talking, the woman sitting across the table from us leaned forward on her forearms, palms flattened against the surface, attentive to every word. Her husband sat behind her and to the left, leaning back in his chair, his face without emotion.

As Lloyd was finishing, she suddenly lifted her right arm above her head and pounded her fist against the table as she spoke the words forever etched in my mind:

"Never! Never, have I heard words like this come from the mouth of a man! I want to read that book right now!"

Lloyd looked over at her husband and said, "Well, Sir, what do you think?"

He leaned further back in his chair and, after a brief pause, said, "It's all right, for now."

As the three of us prepared for bed, we marveled at God's grace and how He is always at work drawing us to Him. It reminded us that these medical missions are more than just providing medical care. They are about being small "hope-givers," just as Christ is our big "Hope-giver," to a hurting world in need of hope. The next day, we gave her a Bible in Russian.

CHAPTER 71

Sharing Their Stories

In the book *The Insanity of God*, the author recounts his time as an American missionary in Somalia during the late 1980s through the early 1990s, a time when perhaps no place on earth was more filled with suffering, hardship, and death. It was truly "Hell on earth."

The missionary and his small team risked their lives with every trip into this desolate land. There was no order, no law, except those imposed by the two warring factions. It was a world of total chaos, where men, women, and children were either starving by the thousands or caught in the crossfire of the brutal civil war around them.

Increasingly frustrated by their inability to help in any truly meaningful way, the missionary reflected, *"The people I wanted to help were living in such horrible conditions that my natural response was to focus only on what they lacked."*

His encounters often began like this:

"Do you need food? We have food. Is your baby sick? We have medicine. Do your children need clothes? We have clothes for them."

But over time, he realized those were not the most important questions. When he finally took the time to truly *listen*, the people themselves told him what they needed most.

He recalled one conversation vividly:

"One day, I asked a bent-over, shriveled woman, 'Tell me what you need most. What can I do for you first?' She looked ancient, but she may have only been in her forties. She began to share her story with me:

I grew up in a village many days from here. My father was a nomad who sold camels and sheep. I married a camel herder who did the same work. He was a good man. Together we had a good life and four children. Then the war came. The militia marched through our village, stealing or slaughtering most of our animals. When my husband tried to stop them from taking our last camel, they beat him. They put a gun to his head...'

(Tears began to trickle down her cheeks.)

I worked hard to care for my children, but then the drought came. Despite everything I tried, it wasn't enough. My oldest boy got sick and died. When the last of our food was nearly gone, my children and I began walking. I hoped that life would be better in the city. But it is not, it is harder. Men with guns are everywhere. They raped and beat me. They took my older daughter. I only have the little one left.'

This woman, like countless others, desperately needed more than what the missionary team had come to offer. Eventually, the writer came to understand a profound truth: what people in pain want most is *not* just food, shelter, or medicine. They want someone, anyone, to *listen*.

This is the power of human presence.

It is never enough to simply feed, clothe, and medically treat the body. When people have endured unspeakable evil, heartbreaking loss, or deep suffering, they often lose all sense of their own *humanity*.

The author continued:

"By listening to their stories, we were telling them that they mattered. We were saying they were important enough to be heard. Just by listening, we could help restore a measure of humanity. Often, that felt more important and more transformative than a dose of life-saving medicine or another day's worth of food."

We are fortunate that we do not live in such a hellish nightmare. But I believe that what this missionary came to understand is equally relevant in our own lives and professions.

Our patients come to us sick and afraid, sometimes dying. They feel vulnerable, often helpless. Their lives have become chaotic. In this increasingly technical and impersonal age of medicine, they can feel that their own humanity has been lost.

But they have *stories*, too.

Their stories may not be as tragic as the one above, but they are still meaningful—perhaps deeply so. All of us are made up of stories. Stories are how we tell others who we are, what we've survived, what we need, what we fear, and what brings us joy.

In the busyness of the day, when it feels like there's not enough time to do *one more thing*, or when you've done all you know to do and still it's not enough, may we choose to sit down with them. May we choose to listen.

Share their stories.

In doing so, we bring the *human side* back into medicine.

And isn't that why we chose this profession in the first place?

CHAPTER 72

Gloom Period

I lay in my bed, tears tracing my face. I struggled to hold them back, my emotions churning like waves in troubled water. The ageless, rust-pocked gray radiator beneath the windows groaned as it emanated chapping, dry heat, static electricity waiting for that first touch. Cold crept under, over, and around the edges of the two single-pane windows with their years of layered paint peeling and cracking; a water-filled tin can hung off the right side. Through the darkness, I surveyed my spartan room, a faint light traversing the room's windows that looked out over the central area of Old South Barracks, the iconic clock standing tall in the middle. No pictures or decorations of any type were allowed; no miscellaneous items scattered about—everything in its proper place. It all seemed surreal. What was happening to me?

It had been six months since I entered the United States Military Academy at West Point, and though I missed my family, I had not experienced anything like this. I had just returned that day from my home in Alabama after a much-anticipated and much-needed Christmas break. As the return to my "Rock-bound Highland home" and five more months of "Plebe Hell" loomed closer, a dread deep inside of me began growing. The dread enveloped me, pressing down like a weighted blanket; oppressive, smothering. There was no light at the end of the proverbial tunnel. For me, there were "infinity and a butt" days until the end of Plebe Year. I could not envision graduation ever coming. It was too distant. Infinity is a long time. My first Term End Exams, looming ahead, added to the dread. Everything was gray, dark, cold. Everyone around me looked miserable. I was living one day at a time. I was in survival mode. I felt hopeless.

What I had not anticipated was how the physical environment would affect me, the short days and long nights of winter; the cold, snow, sleet, and freezing rain; the grayish tint of a low January sun dispersed through the gray clouds and weighted fog, casting dark, long shadows on the Gothic granite structures that are West Point. The endless standing at attention in formations, shivering, the cold sweeping off the frozen Hudson River, its surrounding mountains bluish-gray, leafless, silhouetted against the sky; the cold penetrated layers of heavy wool uniforms and overcoats. The coarse wool pants rubbed the hairs off the upper thighs. Traipsing to class across the icy concrete, your left hand and arm carrying your books and ever-present slide rule, right hand always ready to salute. It was a world of gray; gray stone, gray clouds, gray uniforms; a world of dampness and cold; a world of rules, regulations, and routines. It was a hard, demanding world, testing me to my limits, demanding my all. I was miserable.

I missed Saturday nights with my older brother, Michael, watching Johnny Carson and sharing pizza. I missed eating like a normal person, not sitting at attention on the front edge of your seat, eyes fixed on the West Point Crest at the top of the plate, taking tiny two-chew-and-swallow-only bites, ordering arms after every bite, while being harassed by a warped-minded second classman. I missed my mother's lasagna and oatmeal cookies. I missed doing nothing! Quitting was not an option, though. I had to persevere, and I drew strength knowing I was not alone. I had my classmates. We were a *band of brothers*. We were there for each other. I cherished that special bond, and that made all the difference.

Nearly fifty years have passed since I first reported to the *Man in the Red Sash* on a hot July 2nd day in 1973 and began the unique 47-month West Point experience. Those first six months marked the beginning of my *rite of passage* from a 17-year-old boy to the Army officer and man I wanted to become. The Gloom Period played an unexpected yet important role in my passage.

CHAPTER 73

"This Is Me!"

He reminded me of a Pit Bull, this sometimes cantankerous but always fascinating World War II veteran. We first met in 1992, shortly after I arrived in Burlington, North Carolina, following my years in the Army. Chronologically, he was in his early 70s, but physiologically, he was years younger. Square-jawed, short and stocky with broad shoulders and muscular, tattooed arms, I could easily envision a once physically imposing, rakishly handsome young man.

For over 20 years, I listened to his "movie script" life, punctuated by adventure, exotic travel, and unspeakable danger. As he reached his 90s, his mind remained sharp, but his body was failing. Yet the stories continued, and I became increasingly enamored with them. These were stories that needed to be heard lest they be forgotten. Each one was created over a lifetime, like a beautiful tapestry woven painstakingly, each stitch reflecting a moment in time.

I admit I was initially dubious of his stories. They seemed too exciting, too adventurous, and too dangerous to be true. After all, he was just an "old man." What could he have done? I knew better than to default to that presumptuous position, so I kept asking questions. I wanted to hear and absorb his stories.

From the Bronx of New York City, he had been a state champion Golden Glove boxer and a gymnast, later even becoming a circus acrobat. He held an array of jobs: skyscraper construction, bar bouncer, traveling salesman, and eventually a successful businessman. It was his life in the Navy, though, of which movies are made and books written.

He was an original Navy frogman, the predecessor to the current Navy SEALs. In the early morning darkness, hours before the bloody carnage that would be D-Day, June 6, 1944, he led a team of frogmen ashore on the coast of France. Their purpose: to "quietly and quickly" secure critical bridgeheads, all closely guarded by the enemy. They did so using only a knife. They could not risk alerting others.

He told the story in a matter-of-fact, this-was-what-I-was-trained-to-do way. There was no bragging, no regret. Yet as he spoke, he seemed distant, remembering.

How he loved to talk about the women he had known during those years! He claimed to have had a proverbial "girlfriend in every port." This seemed too scripted to be true. Then I had an epiphany. Did he have any photographs of these women and, more importantly, of himself, that he would be willing to share with me? He immediately answered that he did—an entire album filled with pictures from his war days and of his "girlfriends." That did it. I asked him to bring the album to his next visit.

He proudly carried in an old, leather-bound, dusty album. There he was, in black and white, young, handsome, strong, the physique of a champion boxer, gymnast, and warrior, just as his stories had portrayed. In one picture, his arms were around his "Band of Brothers," head cocked sideways, a mischievous grin on his face.

With awe, I turned each page, his youth frozen in time. He took the album and opened it to the latter half, and there before me appeared the women from his stories, beautiful in their youth yet slowly fading in those stills. Arms intertwined, faces smiling agelessly, a lifetime ahead of them. I counted over 30 pictures from around the world.

The pictures cried out, "This is me! I was young once! I did many things, even great things! I have stories to tell; listen to me; I still matter!"

I closed the album, overwhelmed with emotion; awe, respect, admiration, humbled that he would share this with me. I felt ashamed that I had failed to "see" all my patients for who they once were: young, vibrant, with an unknown future ahead, waiting to make their difference in the world.

May the words "This is me!" resonate within you and allow you to see patients not in the black and white of old, fading pictures, but in the "living color" that was their life. Let us not forget that they were young once and have stories we need to hear.

CHAPTER 74

A Little Moment of Joy

The cab driver pulled up to a small house, typical of the post–WWII era. He honked his horn and waited. He honked a second time, but no one came. He contemplated leaving, as it was near the end of his shift, but decided to go knock on the door. Through the door, he heard a voice and something scraping across the floor. The door slowly opened, and a frail, elderly woman, with several suitcases at her side, stood before him. She appeared to be in her 90s. There was a noticeable sadness about her.

She thanked him for coming as he helped her down the steps to the taxi. He asked where she wanted to go, and she quietly responded, "To the Hospice Home." She explained that her doctor had told her she had less than six months to live. She had no family left to care for her. Her husband had died a few years before.

Suddenly she said, "Could you take me downtown?" Hesitantly, knowing it was out of the way, he agreed. He drove slowly through the town where she had lived her entire life. She was seeing it for the last time. Her eyes glistening, she reminisced of times long ago, the building where she had her first job, the park where her husband first kissed her, the matinee theater, dance hall, soda shop... her children.

After two hours, they arrived at the Hospice Home. She asked how much she owed. With tears in his eyes, he turned off the meter and told her there was no charge. Helping her into a waiting wheelchair, she thanked him again and said, "You gave an old woman a little moment of joy."

I read the above story on social media and was deeply moved. We often care for those nearing the end of their lives. It is so easy to see them as just another old person with their myriad of physical problems, increasingly dependent upon others. We forget that once they were young, vibrant, strong, navigating life as best they could. They have their own stories. Where did they grow up? What did they do for a living? Simple questions that could open unexpected windows, allowing glimpses into their lives and hearts.

I always asked my older male patients whether they had served in the military. Many of my most memorable stories came from that question. History came to life—Pearl Harbor, Guadalcanal, Tarawa, Iwo Jima, Omaha Beach, the Battle of the Bulge, the 8th Air Force over Germany, Chosin Reservoir, Ia Drang—bloody places, costly places, still very much alive in the recesses of their minds. I treasured these stories. In their telling, you could see a glimmer in their eyes, hear the pride in their voices, and, for a moment, see them as they once were: young, strong, their entire life ahead of them.

Each of us can give "a little moment of joy" to others. In doing so, we are reminded of the human side of medicine. The rewards can be life-giving to you and to the person telling their stories. Stories are powerful. They need to be heard lest they be lost forever.

Who will you bring "a little moment of joy" to today?

CHAPTER 75

The Potter's Hands

In her book *In Shock*, Dr. Rana Awdish, an intensivist, describes how, after a near-death experience and prolonged, difficult recovery, she came to appreciate the importance that people have had in her life. She spoke of those who trained her and of her colleagues, each playing a role in molding her, like clay in a potter's hands, into who she was. She said, "I learned from them that relationships can shape us... that we can allow ourselves to be supported by an enveloping mold in the hands of others."

All of us have had people be our "potter's hands." After my father, the biggest influence was my Little League baseball coach, "Skip." He had been a professional baseball player, but a severe wound from the Korean War ended his career. He turned his passion for baseball on us. His love for the game was contagious. He taught us how to look and to play like a Major Leaguer. I loved it. I loved him. I remember at the age of 12 thinking that one day I would coach Little League. I wanted to bring the same fun and joy to kids, and I tried. I coached youth baseball for nearly 20 years, even before I had children.

There were others as well:

My 11th-grade chemistry teacher, the best teacher in the school. If you could make a "B" in his class, he would write a letter of recommendation to college for you. He taught me how to study.

My high school ROTC instructor. He told me in the 10th grade that, if I got into West Point, which he made clear he doubted, he did not think I would survive the rigorous four years there. He was the only person ever to tell me I could not succeed at something. His words were like a blacksmith stoking a fire, fueling it, making it grow hotter, more powerful. I was determined to prove him wrong.

My Tactical Officer at West Point. A highly decorated combat veteran in Vietnam who became a four-star general. He was the toughest of all the officers assigned to develop, teach, and discipline cadets. There was an intense love-hate relationship between my company mates and him. He made our lives miserable, but secretly we took pride in being in the hardest of the 36 companies there. He taught me physical and mental toughness, perseverance, accountability, responsibility, and attention to detail.

My hospital Commanding Officer in Saudi Arabia during the First Gulf War. His reputation as the toughest Chief of Surgery in the Army Medical Corps preceded him. I know because I trained where he was the Chief and heard all the "stories" from my surgical contemporaries. However, when war came, and I was his Chief of Medicine, he was one of the best leaders for whom I ever served. He knew how to take care of his people.

Who helped mold you? Who invested in, taught, encouraged, and mentored you? Are you doing the same for those coming behind you? You have a special gift to give: your wisdom and knowledge from years of training and experience. In doing so, you become "the hands of a potter," shaping and molding them into the best they can be. In doing so, you will make a difference in their lives just as others made a difference in yours. In doing so, you can find joy.

CHAPTER 76

Fire Pit Time

The flames flicker, tantalizingly reaching upward, and I sit mesmerized. How many times have I sat by my backyard fire pit and watched this ageless dance? I think, I meditate, I pray; a cigar and bourbon often accompany me. I especially love to stand by it while the snow falls, enveloping me in all its beauty. The memories are many, and they are good.

My sons are with me around the pit. I cherish these times. I try to remember every moment, for I know they are numbered, the passage of time unrelenting. Our conversations vary, often deep, always important. I learn their hearts and, better yet, they learn mine. I am happy and so very proud.

I am with friends, my "Band of Brothers", fellow physicians with whom I have served through the years. With cigar and bourbon in hand, we, too, talk about "anything and every-thing," sometimes medical, most often not. I sit in awe of them as I ponder the lives they have touched and, more, the differ-ence they have made. We are growing old together. It is good to have such friends. I love them as my own brothers.

I sit surrounded by young faces—the heart of the medical staff, those who are coming behind me, their "yet to come" of the future still greater than their "already been" of the past. They are my passion, the real reason I have remained in medicine for as long as I have. I want to invest in, teach, encourage, and mentor them in any way I can. They are the future leaders of medicine: the visionaries, the decision-makers, the catalysts behind the inevitable changes that must come if we are to provide the best for those entrusting their care, often their lives, to us. They want someone to mentor them.

Often, it is an unspoken request, conveyed through a language unique to each of them. I have learned to "hear" the subtleties of this language through my years of leading medical missions and teaching medical students, PAs, and NPs. I want to be there for them, so I make myself available. I do so around the fire pit as often as possible. We share food, drink, and life-giving conversation. Relationships are made and strengthened between different specialties, and trust is created. Only trust can bond them together so they can be the unified, cohesive, and effective team required to lead us forward. "Fire pit time" brings them together, and that brings me joy.

Medicine demands much from us, and we need much in return. We all need our own "fire pit time," however that may look. I hope you will find yours.

CHAPTER 77

Every Patient Every Time

She began telling me the same "sob story," but this time I looked at her and coldly said, "Mrs. ___, you are going home. I don't care what you have to say, you are leaving today. I need the bed for someone else." She began crying. I walked out without saying another word and wrote the discharge order. The intern with me said the words I will always remember: "Man, what you just did was cruel." I looked at him and said, "I don't care. I'm tired, we need the bed, and she is going home." The hard reality is that at that moment, I did not care.

It was the second year of my Internal Medicine training at one of the Army's busiest hospitals. I was finishing 15 months of inpatient work; no days off, no limitations on the hours worked. The patient had metastatic breast cancer. She had been ready to go home for at least a couple of days but kept begging me tearfully not to send her, saying she was not ready. By that time, I was completely exhausted emotionally, mentally, and physically. Always, like a black cloud hanging over me, there was the never-ending pressure to discharge patients so more could be admitted. There were always more patients.

We all know what it's like to be pushed to our emotional and physical limits with long hours, never-ending sick patients, and the ensuing stress of being responsible for their care, ultimately, their life. I vividly remember those days and reaching the point of no longer seeing patients as people in need of care, but rather as "more work." Another case of congestive heart failure, stroke, pneumonia, sepsis—you can fill in the blank. The patient simply became a faceless name on the door, another diagnosis taking up more of my precious time.

This can happen to any of us if we do not guard ourselves against it. We need to remind ourselves why we went into medicine. We need to see each patient as a person in need of help, vulnerable and frightened by the unknown, having to trust us for their care. It is easy, in the busyness of our work, to forget this: to forget that they are someone's loved one, deeply cared for and loved. It's easy to forget that, no matter their condition, they are still deserving of our best effort and most compassionate care, to be treated with kindness, respect, and dignity. Every patient, every time.

As always, thank you for all you do every day for those who place their trust in you.

CHAPTER 78

We Are Right Here With You

My Daddy died peacefully on March 14, 2018, in his home of 46 years, with his family around him. He was 87 years old. A 14-day vigil came to an end with his final breath, and our tears that followed. My hero was gone. It's strange to suddenly realize that with the death of both parents, you are now "next in line" for the inevitable.

The 14 days I was by his side proved to be more emotionally and physically exhausting than I could have imagined. Every day, I was sure it would be his last. We all stayed nearby, lest we not be there when God brought him home. He died as he lived his life. He was a retired Infantry Lieutenant Colonel, having served 22 years in the Army. Prior to this, he served 4 years as a Marine during the Korean War. He was the toughest man I knew. He completed the Army's most demanding training and served two combat tours in Vietnam, earning numerous medals for valor in combat. This same toughness continued to the last. His once physically strong body wasted away to a mere shell. Yet somehow (some reason?), he held on. My brothers and sister lovingly told him it was okay to let go and be with God and Mama, just in case he needed that permission to leave us.

What do you say or do during these times? We did all we could to keep him comfortable, and Hospice was a godsend. I found myself standing at the head of his bed, stroking his bald head, and saying, "We are right here with you, Daddy." I said this over and over. I wanted to be sure he knew he was not alone. The words came so naturally, without even thinking. As I continued to say these words, it hit me that these exact words, "We are right here with you," were the new brand statement for the hospital system where I worked. Now I understand their true impact. They came from a place deep inside me. They will forevermore carry a deeper, more personal meaning. They are no longer simply well-meaning words to be read or spoken. They are now very personal to me, and because they are, they have become very real to me.

As you care for your patients, I hope these words also become personal to you, and subsequently, the impact you have on their lives will be even greater. May they always be a reminder of the difference you make in the lives of those you serve. Thank you for being right there with them when they need you the most.

CHAPTER 79

The Last Time

The man sat at the front of the drift boat as it wobbled gently, anchored at the river's edge. The flyfishing guide sat behind him, making final preparations for the day's float downriver. He had flyfished for nearly 40 years. He even tied his own flies and made fly rods, but age and unwelcome health problems had slowly brought an end to these. And now, it seemed, to his beloved flyfishing as well.

Something inside him spoke. This was the last time he would be on the river that, long ago, had become a part of him. He tried to explain to others the "oneness" he felt with the river, and with flyfishing too, but few understood. The guide understood, though. They had met years earlier and, though he was still "the guide," he was now much more than that. He was a friend.

Countless conversations on the water, interwoven with countless casts to countless rising trout, had cemented their friendship. He sensed his friend knew this was the last time as well. There was no hurry in the preparation for the trip. Few words were spoken.

A sadness enveloped him, like an early morning mist rising ethereally from the river, the cold water caressed by the warmer air above. This was a tailwater; its beginning was at the bottom of a deep lake held behind a dam, the deepest water maintaining a near-constant coldness. It not only provided electric power to the surrounding area, it gave life to the innumerable Browns and Rainbows that thrived in its waters. Only cold, clean, well-oxygenated water would allow them to survive. The river provided just that, and for the man, even more. He thought back to his first time flyfishing and chuckled to himself. He had no idea what he was doing that day. He only knew that for as long as he could remember, he wanted to learn to flyfish. Where that desire came from, he had no clue. As a young boy, there was a movie, *Spencer's Mountain*, that was a favorite of his. There was a scene in the movie with Henry Fonda and Wally Cox flyfishing while imbibing some forbidden whiskey. They were trying to catch the "big one," Fonda knew lived in that stretch of water. Maybe that was the start? His father wasn't a fisherman, so growing up, he didn't fish as much as he would have liked, but he did whenever he could.

It was a gorgeous late October day, that first time; the trees a tapestry of orange, red, green, and yellow; the sun dancing off the water in all its brilliance. He was so hopeful of catching that first trout.

The hours that followed, however, were spent either untangling a bird's nest of hair-thin line or preparing to tangle with the next attempted cast. He never saw a trout, never had a strike—yet he came off the river happy, determined that he *would* learn to do this. Thanks to someone he met soon after, his apprenticeship began, and with it, a very special friendship.

Brad was in his early 30s and had previously been an Orvis guide. He saw the man's determination to learn, and over the next few years, taught him how to flyfish. Amazingly, Brad never fished when they were together. He simply taught, only using the fly rod to demonstrate how to do something better or to teach something new.

Brad eventually did the same with each of the man's three sons as they became old enough to learn. Precious memories from the years that followed, of backpacking and flyfishing with each of them, returned. His eyes glistened.

As he sat, his friend finishing the final preparations, the cloud of sadness began to lift—just as the mist on the water does with the rising of the sun. If this was *the last time*, then he would take in every moment, basking in the joy that flyfishing had brought him. His memories were enough now.

His friend stepped in the boat, raised the anchor, handed him his fly rod, and the boat began to move.

The man was happy.

CHAPTER 80

The Bugler's Last Note

It will happen to all of us, some sooner than others. Sometimes it comes as a well-wrapped package, years in the making, filled with celebration, affirmation, and anticipation. Other times, though, it's not so neatly tied. Sometimes, it is unexpected, leaving you disheveled, confused, unsure, sad, hurt, and angry; a cauldron of emotions.

It may be thirty years or more in coming, but it *will* come— like the light at the end of that proverbial tunnel; the "not yet" of the future increasingly replaced by the "already been" of the past. The bugler's last note was waiting to be played.

It's the time when you leave the work that, in many ways, has defined who you are, for that "next stage" in life, however it may look. For some, one's identity as a person is threatened, and fear and uncertainty follow. For others, it's an unexplored path that veers off the main road, disappearing into the forest, its ultimate destination unknown. A new adventure beckoning.

As I look back on my life's journey *to make a difference* in this world, there is an exact time and place at which I can say, "That was the start, the beginning, my reveille, my early morning bugle call."

It was July 2, 1973, the day I entered West Point. I was seventeen years old, and I knew, at least I thought I knew, what I wanted to do with my life. I was going to be "an Airborne,

Ranger infantry officer and lead men in combat." But God had other plans for me. Medicine became my calling. Making a difference in the lives of people, my passion.

For over 42 years, I have dedicated my life to serving both my country and others. All things, though, eventually come to an end. General Douglas MacArthur, in his farewell speech to Congress upon his retirement from the Army, eloquently said, *"Old soldiers never die, they just slowly fade away."* And so it is with me.

I do so not so much with sadness, though yes, some sadness is there, but with *extreme gratitude* that I have been able to do what I love most: to care for and serve others, to teach, encourage, and mentor those who follow. I stand now at the edge of that unexplored, untraveled path, poised to take the first step. My "next stage" is waiting. It's how it should be. It's how I want it to be.

It is with sadness, however, that this will be my last *Bugle Note* to you.

Thank you for allowing me to share them with you. I wrote them to encourage you, to support you, and to remind you that what you do is important, what you do makes a difference every day, and what you do, it is still a privilege.

I hope I succeeded in even a small way.

You are appreciated.

You are valued.

You are loved.

Andy Lamb, MD